TELL ME
WHAT
YOU LIKE

TELL ME WHAT YOU LIKE

An Honest Discussion of Sex and Intimacy After Sexual Assault

Katie Simon

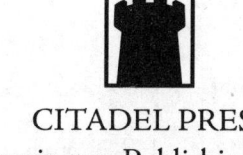

CITADEL PRESS
Kensington Publishing Corp.
kensingtonbooks.com

CITADEL PRESS BOOKS are published by

Kensington Publishing Corp.
900 Third Avenue
New York, NY 10022

All Kensington titles, imprints, and distributed lines are available at special quantity discounts for bulk purchases for sales promotions, premiums, fund-raising, educational, or institutional use. Special book excerpts or customized printings can also be created to fit specific needs. For details, write or phone the office of the Kensington sales manager: Kensington Publishing Corp., 900 Third Avenue, New York, NY 10022, attn Sales Department; phone 1-800-221-2647.

10 9 8 7 6 5 4 3 2 1

First Citadel hardcover printing: August 2025

Printed in the United States of America

ISBN: 978-0-8065-4276-8

ISBN: 978-0-8065-4278-2 (e-book)

Library of Congress Control Number: 2025934267

The authorized representative in the EU for product safety and compliance
is eucomply OU, Parnu mnt 139b-14, Apt 123,
Tallinn, Berlin 11317; hello@eucompliancepartner.com

To the dozens of insightful, resilient, and brave
sexual assault survivors who lent their voices
to this collective narrative. This book would not
exist without you, and now it exists, for you.

Contents

Introduction: We Want More Stories   1

Chapter 1   First, Safety   9

Chapter 2   Check In with Yourself   33

Chapter 3   We Heal in Community   59

Chapter 4   What You Want   77

Chapter 5   To Tell or Not to Tell   87

Chapter 6   First Times   113

Chapter 7   Survivors on Consent   131

Chapter 8   Triggers and Turn-Ons   147

Chapter 9   Pain, Pleasure, and (Optional) Orgasms   173

Chapter 10   Overcoming Setbacks   187

Aftercare: The Future of Sex   209

Resources   217

Acknowledgments   220

Endnotes   222

Index   225

Introduction:
We Want More Stories

IN THE MONTHS after a man raped me, I walked past shelves in bookstore after bookstore, furtively glancing at book spines out of the corner of my eye. I was searching not so much for a book as for answers to a burning question: How could I ever have sex again after being raped? I wondered if I would find anybody willing to "deal with" my issues, and what "dealing with" those issues might look like. I had a deeper question, too, which I felt but couldn't articulate: Would I ever experience sexual pleasure again? It's been over a decade since I started looking for the answers to these questions, for the stories like the ones in this book. I didn't know it then, but I know now: It's not just me who's looking.

Even today, post-#MeToo movement, discussions around sex after sexual assault are largely absent from public discourse. The topic is not often addressed in sexual abuse healing guides, sexual assault recovery therapy, or PTSD treatment. Google "sex after sexual assault," and the pickings are sparse, singular, and surface level. We're only just beginning to reckon with the impact sexual assault has on its survivors. There's an urgent issue that we've barely addressed, because it lies at the still taboo intersection of two subjects: sex and sexual assault. The only aspect we're talking about is a fresh definition of consent, especially legally, which is not so much about sex as it is about safety. We're not talking about bigger picture issues, like how the #MeToo movement itself and the subsequent news cycles are impacting our sex lives. While many individuals escape assault, we are collectively affected by the threat of violation, collectively impacted

1

by the rise in stories about sexual assault, collectively challenged by behavior that perpetuates rape culture. It's not just sexual assault survivors who are wondering: Where do we go from here?

After experiencing sexual abuse as a child, I struggled to explore my sexuality as a teenager. Eventually, I became sexually active—until, when I was eighteen, a stranger raped me. A month after the rape, before I'd told anybody or even thought about resources that might help me, I made out with an acquaintance. I knew I was doing it to erase and write over what had happened. I clung to his lips like an oxygen mask underwater. At the same time, I wondered if wanting sex, if acting on my desire, had led to the rape. I didn't know that all of my thoughts and actions were normal, or that this process of trial and error was how most survivors navigated sex post-assault. I didn't know that it would be more than a year before my next kiss, almost two years before I let another person undress me.

I went to therapy in those intervening years. At first I didn't even know what trauma was: the emotional and physiological distress that follows an unspeakably painful experience. Once I found my footing, my therapist and I went through seemingly every aspect of rape recovery: trust, self-esteem, soothing panic responses, recovering rational thought. However, we never broached how sex might be different for me now because of my trauma history. I was left with unarticulated questions. How might my history, especially the recent rape, impact my desires, my self-worth in romantic relationships, my sexuality? How might my views on consent, masturbation, and casual sex change? I knew sexual assault affected all this and more, but how, too, did other pre- and post-trauma factors play into my sexual present?

As therapy wound down, I started seeing David. Because it was not something that came up in therapy, I still navigated sex with him mostly through trial and error. I paid the most attention to what the cultural conversation told me was important: consent. I was so focused on consent, on boundaries—essentially, on trying to prevent another rape—that I decentered my own pleasure during sexual experiences. I considered sex that left me safe but unsatisfied to be "good"—if not the goal. I put thought into what communication I wanted and into making sure I was with a partner who would respect my boundaries. It was my first brush with a bigger lesson: the "rules" of sex and relationships popular today can prove less important to sexual assault survivors, who must deal with the impact that trauma has on us. At the time, I thought my experience was mine alone. It would be years before I realized that what I felt in isolation was actually normal. Part of my drive to write this book was to introduce a new lexicon, similar to the dissemination of therapy-speak: the language of trauma-sensitive dating, which anybody can learn.

Something else made its way into my considerations, slowly but surely: my body. Sex for a survivor can lead to unpleasant outcomes, including a panic response; avoidance, or removing oneself from the situation; dissociation, or feeling mentally disconnected from one's body; and attempting to please one's partner out of rational or irrational fears. Fight or flight; freeze and appease. For me, sex often led to a trapped, frozen panic response. Tens of millions of people across the United States experience sexual assault, and 94 percent of survivors experience symptoms of traumatic stress.[1] These symptoms, such as decreased trust, anxiety, powerlessness, and depression, may affect our sex lives. While the experience of panicking is in itself disruptive, for me, it opened up another can of worms: explaining my panic in a way that might yield a healthy response from my partner. It's difficult to talk about the symptoms of PTSD and the fallout of trauma without talking about the details of the trauma itself.

It was through eventually finding a compassionate sex partner that I learned what I needed from one. But, in today's challenging sexual climate, not all of us come across a partner who responds in the way we hope. In fact, a less-than-compassionate sex partner may have led you to search, like me, for a book that addresses these struggles. Many of us don't really know what to look for in the people we have sex with, especially when it comes to navigating trauma. If our sexual partners aren't as in sync as we'd like them to be, and our therapists are skirting the subject, the only way to navigate sex post-assault is by learning from the experiences of other survivors. It's difficult to broach the topic of one's own sexual assault, but perhaps even more difficult to discuss the impact of trauma on one's sex life. Yet keeping these conversations behind closed doors can actually harm the tens of millions of people with trauma histories.

Years into our relationship, my decision to break up with David was not easy—ending any long-term relationship comes with doubts—but it was made more difficult and complicated by my lingering, trauma-related fears about sex, trust, and self-worth. I later learned, through my research and interviews, that it's common to feel a breakup is tied to a long past trauma. In a way, I was back at square one: I had to relearn how to have sex with somebody new—and thus put myself at risk, in the hands of somebody who might not know how to respond to my sexual issues, or who might even assault me again. Though many people face challenges when it comes to their sex lives, for sexual assault survivors, "bad" sex (either emotionally or physically)—even if it's consensual—may trigger a panic attack or some other negative reaction a nonsurvivor wouldn't experience.

In a way, sleeping with new people, with more people, was the beginning of my research for this book. Sex became something I could shape positively, not just seek safety in. My relationship with David, and subsequent casual relationship with my friend James, made me feel heard, my body feel safe. David not only waited months into our relationship to have sex with me, he encouraged me to take my time. James checked in about my comfort level, made no big deal about stopping at any time, and was always available to listen when I felt upset. I'm sure that both of them felt frustrated or upset about my reactions at times, but they centered my needs and understood that the foundation of healthy, satisfying sex for both of us was the assurance that I would feel comfortable. At the time, I didn't realize how unusual David's or James' reactions were. I had taken for granted that all people would be as compassionate as my ex-boyfriend and recent fuckbuddy; I was unprepared for the man who would make me leave not just his bed, but his apartment building, when I had a panic attack.

Dating forced me to wrestle with the rape I experienced as a teenager, but it also made me face the prolonged sexual abuse I experienced as a child, at the hands of a girl I trusted. The abuse made me associate other women's bodies with danger and pain. But after puberty, I noticed my growing attraction to women. Female friends kissed me, and while they were probably playing around, I couldn't keep my heart from racing, my body from wanting more. But a sick feeling would bubble up in my stomach, confusion erupting inside me: How could I be attracted to another girl when a girl hurt me? The therapy I struggled through in childhood never treated that abuse as trauma, and it was easier to fall into heteronormative expectations than face that abuse head-on, questioning how it might affect my willingness to explore my sexuality—or enact it at all. I buried every feeling I had toward a woman before it could develop into something more than a crush. As a teenager, a few negative reactions to my disclosure of my sexuality as something other than straight ended up keeping me in the closet for years.

In my midtwenties, after years of trauma therapy addressing the rape at age eighteen and the earlier childhood abuse, I came out as queer to a handful of friends and family. I received mixed reactions—mostly confusion over why it took me so long to disclose this. As I would discover over the course of my research, my sexual orientation was difficult for me to embrace because of the identity of the person who abused me. When considering coming out, I imagined feeling obligated to answer questions about why it had taken me so long. Answering honestly would mean disclosing my history of abuse, and it took years to feel comfortable enough to be so open. Not only could I face negative consequences for coming out and disclosing my trauma history, but I also stood to lose out on the chance for the best-case scenario, being openly queer and embraced for it. The stakes felt high.

There is no single narrative in the trajectory of survivors' sex lives. The process of healing is just as varied as any individual's sexual growth. In order to better understand survivors' sex lives, we need to look past the superficial way we view the healing process. Our society too often defines "recovery" and "healing" as terms that imply being freed from trauma—to somehow live as if the trauma never happened. But for many survivors, recovery and healing mean something else entirely: an integration of the impact of trauma into our lives and an acceptance of how it has changed us and how we have grown in its wake. "Post-traumatic growth" as a concept suggests that while sexual violation does not necessarily have meaning, we can find meaning through how we choose to repair ourselves in its aftermath.

Like so many other survivors, my familial history, relationships, and upbringing affected my journey toward post-traumatic growth. Before they fled during the genocidal pogroms against Jews in Ukraine, members of my family were publicly whipped, tortured, murdered—and forced to witness and fall victim to mass rape. There is increasing conversation about intergenerational violence in the United States, and when it comes to twenty-first-century rape culture, I think we face a related issue: intergenerational silence. I am the first person in my family to speak openly about sexual trauma. Breaking my silence was one of the most difficult—and most healing—aspects of my post-traumatic growth. Once I did, I was able to navigate my sex life with a strong enough voice to keep me feeling safe and, eventually, to experience authentic pleasure and joy.

Although I've been writing as long as I can remember, I didn't find an audience until I started writing about my experiences of violence. I didn't just write about violence, however; more frequently, I wrote about how sexual assault and rape affected my sex life. I wrote about what the #MeToo movement means for sexual pleasure, what disclosing trauma histories means in the bedroom, what a world that too often defends powerful offenders could be if we instead attuned ourselves to nuanced survivor narratives. I started getting emails, Instagram DMs, and Facebook messages from readers telling me my words were resonating. Without asking, I began to hear these other survivors' stories of sex after sexual assault—some similar, some vastly different—from mine. Many of them told me they had never spoken about this with anyone else before. Their stories were not being told.

I decided to start interviewing survivors about their experiences. I expected these stories to be triggering. Instead, I found them steadying. Hearing about survivors' sex lives normalized my own, even when our experiences and identities were not aligned.

I also realized I had been right. My story was one of many, a single voice in a chorus. In order to paint a fuller and more accurate picture, I needed to bring these other voices into the conversation. I have had mostly positive experiences telling partners about my assaults; many of my interviewees have not (if they've chosen to disclose at all). I avoid physical pain during sex; many of my interviewees seek it out. My definition of consent involves plenty of straightforward verbal communication; many people prefer systems built on safewords or body language cues. Our stories are different because other areas of our identities are different. Though I have mental disabilities, I do not have physical ones. I am nonbinary, queer, and Jewish; many survivors are none of these things. My stories are a tiny fraction of the collective experience of sexual assault survivors. If my end goal is to tell stories that more survivors can identify with—to broaden the representation—in order to make us all feel less alone, I have to go beyond my own. It wasn't my personal experience of sex after sexual assault that catalyzed me to write this book. It was realizing that my personal experience was not representative, not universal. Over the course of dozens of interviews on this topic, I have yet to hear from a survivor who hasn't experienced trauma's impact on their sex life. And while some voices are missing from this book, those gaps largely reflect potential interviewees' discomfort with talking about these still-taboo subjects and speak to the self-selecting nature of interview-based research. There are as many stories as there are survivors, but I believe you, like me, will connect with stories of people with vastly different lived experience from your own. We have all been through violence, and we all seek safety in our sexual selves.

This book is for survivors, not just about us. Shaped by real survivors' real stories, I made the choice early on not to amplify the voices of subject matter experts over or even alongside survivors', because survivors' stories don't need outside validation to have meaning and substance. At times, this book includes research or expert perspectives for context or to explain psychological concepts. But there are plenty of resources to learn about PTSD, sex therapy, or trauma research. The real experts on the experience of sex after sexual assault are survivors ourselves. Our stories, our voices, are what's missing from the conversation.

Our voices are not just a conversation within the survivor community. This book normalizes a range of post-assault sexual experiences, while driving home the reality that many people having sex today are survivors of sexual assault. These stories are survivors', but the broader picture they paint is for anybody seeking more intentional, connected, and pleasurable sex—with the knowledge that rape culture impacts sex for everyone. This book isn't meant to be particularly hopeful or uplifting, because it seeks to expose the reality of what is happening in survivors' real lives, which is messy—and not discussed enough. In place of hope, this book seeks to create community, a compendium of voices so that none of us have to feel alone.

This book tackles the obstacles a survivor might face while rebuilding a sex life after sexual trauma: dissociation, panic attacks, physical pain, flashbacks, and more. Each chapter includes a varied selection of survivors' stories in order to normalize and uplift a diversity of healing experiences. Each story also ties in a topic of broad interest, such as embodied consent, media perceptions of sexual assault survivors, sexual regret, and how to have vulnerable conversations with a partner. These stories illuminate how survivors have navigated their struggles into positive practices and outlooks, reimagining what sex can look like—not only for survivors, but for all of us.

Although the survivors' stories I've heard vary greatly, I've identified with parts of all of them. If nothing else, I've found myself nodding along with almost every survivor's answer to the question on which I ended our interviews: "What resources would be most helpful when dealing with sexual assault's impact on your sex life?"

They almost unanimously gave the same answer: We want more stories.

The survivors in these pages have told their stories. Not just, as is common, about the worst things that have happened to us, but also about the best. When I've struggled to work on this book, I've returned over and over again to what so many survivors have shared with me, beacons in the night. Every part of this book seeks to normalize our experiences and light the path forward.

This book didn't exist after a man raped me. So, I decided to write it.

CHAPTER 1

First, Safety

THE STORY OF HOW to get better may not start with the first positive step. Sometimes, it starts with recognizing the circumstances that prevent us from taking a step forward at all. This chapter includes the stories of people who became stuck in cycles of domestic violence, details why and how they left, and untangles the impact prolonged exposure to violence had on their eventual healing—underscoring the importance of leaving an abusive situation. Intimate partner violence can affect people of any sexual orientation or gender, from any background. The threat of violence is always reason enough to leave, and the impact of prolonged exposure (which can turn into complex post-traumatic stress disorder) makes it even harder to heal when safety is eventually secured.

But this chapter isn't just for people dating their abusers—it's for anybody who feels threatened in their day-to-day life, and for whom that threat might hinder healing. The threat can be individual, cultural, or communal. It's not just physical danger that gets in the way of recovery. Psychological distress from past or present trauma can be just as debilitating. In this chapter, survivors detail the most helpful social and psychological support they received that enabled them to leave an abusive relationship or toxic environment and find stable ground. Most importantly, this chapter is a jumping-off point for readers. In order for the rest of the book to be constructive, a baseline of physical and psychological safety must be established. You don't have to be dating a rapist for rape culture to take hold of your life.

Sitting on a couch across from my new therapist, I was attempting to describe why I was so upset that a man I barely knew had rejected me. It wasn't much of a loss. We weren't close and had only been out a couple of times. "He felt safe to me," I said.

"What do you mean by that word, 'safe'?" she asked. I clasped my hands together in my lap. The truth was, I wasn't sure how to describe what I meant by that. My last relationship had been abusive, so I knew what I wasn't looking for. At the time, I didn't realize how much my definition of safe had been shaped over the years to mean somebody who didn't have the red flags that indicated they might become dangerous. Instead of focusing on what I wanted in a partner, I was seeking out the opposite of whatever I was afraid of.

Then and now, I tend to think somebody I'm dating is safe until proven otherwise. It's a survival strategy: If I started at my real baseline, rooted in fear, I'd never go out with anybody. Instead, I'm watchful of signs they could become actively unsafe, and operate under a "wait and see" policy. If somebody feels "safe" to me, it often just means that I trust them subconsciously; maybe they helped me out when something small but painful happened, or they made me feel taken care of. But this flipped mentality—innocent until proven guilty—can lead to an early powerful attachment that isn't necessarily earned. Getting attached early can lead to a lot of rejection, and dating can be painful for me. What another person considers a fling or a casual start to a potential relationship, I see as the first step in a bigger relationship narrative. It's not every time—I have casual sex—but if I like someone and see them as emotionally and physically safe, I tend to end up getting more attached, and rejected, than I probably need to.

On the other hand, sometimes I form powerful negative impressions of people early on and refuse to take into consideration other factors or apologies that could resolve early issues. It's like holding a grudge, but my body takes over and I'm not able to hit override. I have a visceral reaction that prevents me from being open to relationships.

It's not just abusive partners that raise my baseline fear. When trying to date or sleep with someone, I'm also affected by circumstantial factors, like medical issues that cause pain, or triggering news cycles. After the October 7th massacre in Israel, when systematic sexual violence and torture were used as methods of terrorism and livestreamed globally, I had trouble trusting new partners enough to sleep with them. My sex drive was remarkably low, and for a while I only felt comfortable sleeping with Jewish partners, or people I already knew. The aftershock—witnessing global denial of the atrocities—was triggering in its own right, and the feeling of being disbelieved about sexual violence was magnified all over the news and social media. While I had been upset by trauma- and rape-related news cycles in my life in the past, this one hit the closest to home.

I always felt like I was the only one affected by these kinds of questions about safety as central to a post-assault sex life—until I started speaking to other survivors, including those dealing with the aftermath of abusive relationships.

In order to heal, we have to recognize what happened to us. Lexi M., a bisexual woman, sees a lot of fellow survivors minimizing their experiences so they don't seem as severe, trying to shy away from the blunt force of the impact. "We lessen the bar for what we consider assault," she says. The effect of this is not just in not counting assaults for what they are, but in discounting the impact of what happened. Lexi says that survivors don't get to take up space for the fallout—the trauma—of seemingly "lesser" assaults. "A lot of us downplay what happened to us," Lexi says to me. Realistically, she recognizes that she's been sexually assaulted many, many more times by men than she "counts." "A man walked up to me in a bar and slapped my ass," Lexi remembers. "I did not know him, I did not consent to it, and he was just like 'With an ass like that, you should be a stripper.'" Lexi sees what happened as a sexual assault but knows that many people see these kinds of experiences as "just a thing that happens to me when I'm out."

It's not just assaults in public that get minimized. Some interactions Lexi has experienced that are more akin to rape get downplayed, too—the whole spectrum gets downplayed: "Everything feels less serious than it actually is." Lexi remembers what a former partner said when she explained the full extent of the assaults she has experienced: "Well, that can't be considered sexual assault 'cause, then, like, everyone will have been sexually assaulted, or everyone will have sexually assaulted someone." She looks at me and shakes her head in frustration, and remembers thinking how close he was to actually getting the point.

Lexi has noticed that to many people, for something to be traumatizing, it has to be "really bad." But that's not how you define traumatic. "Our body," she explains, "has a very large nervous system reaction to something that is scary, harmful, upsetting—whatever. And then, because of that, moving forward, our nervous system has disproportionately large reactions based off of that initial traumatic moment." As Lexi points out, trauma is the response to a traumatic event, not just the experiencing of that event. Trauma is the fallout after something terrible happens and our physiological response to the triggering event gets stuck in the present. Trauma is not feeling safe even after the traumatic event has passed.

However, sometimes we aren't able to access a sense of safety, not because of trauma symptoms, but because we *are not* safe. That may mean recognizing that we are trapped in an abusive, violent relationship, or acknowledging we live in a world that is threatening to people who appear a certain way in public, or noticing how triggers are baked into the world around us. Locating a sense of safety is impossible if that safety is conditional on another person's behavior; we need to generate our own safety in order for it to be sustainable. If you're trapped in an unsafe situation, whether that's with an abusive partner or another source of prolonged discomfort, your body won't be able to calm down, and you won't be able to feel safe even if you eventually are in a safe situation.

It's not just abusive partners or physical danger that threaten our well-being and safety and make healing difficult. Survivors I spoke to felt powerless to leave abusive situations, even when they weren't dating their assailants. It can be difficult, if not impossible, to escape an abuser that is a professor of a class you're required to take, or your boss at a job you need, or the coach of a team you've worked hard to make. Some survivors choose to leave these situations, even if it means upending their lives, to prioritize safety.

Psychological distress makes healing difficult, too. A college friend, a gay asexual man, once told me about living through a particularly loud news cycle about a prominent rape trial. Ultimately, he turned off the TV and cried into his partner's shoulder for hours. Sex was off the table for months. When another friend, a straight woman, hears a rape joke, her sex drive plummets for days. Jennifer, a straight woman, describes navigating a world in which she experiences high pressure to drink heavily around potential sex partners. As if that weren't enough, she simultaneously deals with the sexualization of her body as an Asian American woman. When we spoke, she was giving up hope that she could go out to a party or a bar without her body coming under some form of verbal, or even physical, attack. The pressure to drink at times turned into a way out—drinking as anesthetization from a world that simply feels too dangerous to constantly navigate.

Danika Bloom, a straight woman from Canada, explains that much of rape culture there looks the same as in the United States. When she hears politicians making outlandish, damaging claims about pregnancy and rape, it's a lot for her to process as a survivor. If she doesn't have a safe person or a safe space to process that kind of thing, it's hard for Danika to cope and function normally. She may need somebody to not just hold her physically, but also emotionally, intellectually, and spiritually. She needs someone to hold all of her. "There's no stigma around being shot, but there's stigma around being raped. How does that make sense?" Danika asks. That stigma can get in the way of accessing a sense of safety central to healing, whether through preventing a survivor from getting social support or even how a survivor views their own experiences.

Ramona, a demisexual straight woman, brought up how someone else's physical size can be intimidating, especially if they are your partner or potential partner. This is something I think about a lot. I am just over five feet tall. Ramona is five four. When we talked, Ramona shared her experience of meeting with a man who was six seven on a dating app. They spoke online and then on the phone and hit it off, so they agreed to meet in person. Prior to their date, Ramona brought up certain physical boundaries she had, boundaries that she set with all men she dated but that felt particularly important to her in light of their size difference. Rather than understanding that these boundaries were put in place after her sexual assault as a way to protect herself physically and emotionally, he got defensive. His reaction was a huge red flag for Ramona, and she decided not to go on the date after all, but she concedes that his physical size played a role in her decision, too. "I stood no chance against this guy," Ramona tells me, acknowledging her fear that he could simply overpower her. The physical size and strength differences gave her pause, but his behavior made her decision for her. While hyperarousal, or a heightened sense of danger that may or may not correspond with reality, can make survivors feel more threatened, at times the root of hyperarousal is a seed of danger that is worth paying attention to.

Ramona wanted her tall date to say, "I understand that you've been sexually assaulted. I'm so sorry that happened to you. Let me know if I can make you feel more comfortable." Instead, he didn't recognize her needs or the fact that his height might be a legitimate concern for her that he could address and try to ease. Ramona has encountered a similar attitude from men when she points out their racist microaggressions that particularly bother her as a biracial Black woman. They are immediately defensive and unwilling to engage. It can be a form of gaslighting if somebody won't acknowledge the pain you're in, or the way their behavior is toxic or damaging.

Ramona adds that she has done a BDSM session with someone who was very tall, but his overall mannerism was gentle and sweet, and she didn't feel intimidated by him. She finds it's dependent on the person. But at the end of the day, we live in a world that is actually unsafe sometimes, and we have to be careful. Looking out for your own safety isn't a negative thing. Ramona believes that men often think that her boundaries are a judgment of their character, and not about safety, because they don't experience the insecurity that would make them understand. There is an empathy gap.

Many people are given the advice that it's more important to not judge a book by its cover than to prioritize their own safety. We feel like we shouldn't evaluate somebody based on something they can't change, like their size, and that we're being rude by paying attention to our fear. But that's centering the other person's experience, and we need to center our own.

Mason, a bisexual male survivor, is six three and weighs 230 pounds. He recognizes his privilege in almost never feeling physically intimidated by other people. "Someone has to be a real giant for me to feel it," he says. Mason is cautious of how other people perceive his body. "I'm hyperaware of my size," Mason says. He was small as a kid but grew a foot between the ages sixteen and seventeen. This growth spurt changed his perspective, literally, and while he doesn't feel particularly tall or big himself, he's aware of how his body is perceived by others, especially women. "I try to be very careful not to be an intimidating presence physically," Mason says. Rather than writing off women's fears, he chooses to move through space in a more conscious, less threatening way. Mason's self-awareness is refreshing, especially after fruitless conversations I and so many others have had with men urging them to be more conscious of others' personal space.

These threats, which could make anybody feel vulnerable, form particular challenges for survivors attempting to heal from sexual assault and rebuild sex lives we find fulfilling. For some survivors, turning off the TV or avoiding particularly toxic party scenes may be enough to minimize or eliminate the threat. It's important for survivors to take these circumstantial threats seriously and seek out mental and emotional safety, taking measures to regulate our nervous systems and using our skills to minimize the threats' impact.

But sometimes, the threat of rape culture is more menacing than another #MeToo story coming to light or going on a date with somebody who looks scary. Some survivors are still in the process of simply surviving—stuck in abusive relationships or unsafe settings.

Stacey Rose, a straight woman, was a student in her twenties in the Midwest when she began supporting students as a victim advocate through Title IX programs. The work was difficult but fulfilling and set Stacey on her current path as a consent educator.

Meanwhile, Stacey began dating a man. The relationship seemed promising at first, but quickly it devolved into suffocating emotional and sexual abuse. At the same time as Stacey professionally assisted victims of sexual violence, she got trapped in a relationship based on violence. As she worked with survivors, being on call and helping with emergency responses in the middle of the night, she put off recognizing or dealing with abuse happening in her own life. "I was putting other people ahead of myself," Stacey says. While this may seem counterintuitive, it makes a lot of sense when "just leaving" your own abusive context can prove threatening not only to your emotional well-being, but even to your life.

It's easy, from the outside, to judge somebody who gets stuck in a cycle of violence—isn't once enough to leave? When a victim responds differently from our expectations, it can make us uncomfortable. All of a sudden, our definition of assault—something terrible that victims would do anything to prevent from happening again—has been challenged. The narrative we have about what victims do after an assault gets a lot wrong, and it doesn't take into account factors beyond the traumatic event itself. One survivor I spoke to talked about being financially reliant on the partner who was abusing her; he was her only way of accessing housing, and since her family lived thousands of miles away, she felt stranded. Often a repeat abuser tries to isolate their victim socially, discouraging them from trusting friends and family so that we will have less support and be less likely to leave. Plus, an abuser might wait until the relationship is well underway before assaulting their partner, in order to make victims feel even more trapped.

Stacey compartmentalized the abuse in order to function (and work in violence awareness), but it took its toll. Some survivors of domestic violence and abusive relationships may strive to act like they have a "normal" relationship despite the abuse. They introduce their partners to friends, go on vacations together, and spend holidays at each other's family's houses. From the outside, to others, the relationship appears healthy. Often, in retrospect, those same survivors reflect that that drive was just them trying to reclaim power over a relationship that was harmful. We may want to prove to ourselves that we were in control. But Stacey, like other survivors, wasn't. She remained caught in a cycle of violence. Healing in this kind of environment is impossible.

Stacey ultimately came to the decision that she needed to leave her partner, but it wasn't because of the abuse, which felt routine and horribly predictable. Instead, like many people in abusive relationships, she decided to leave because of a "healthy relationship" reason—in her case, learning she had been cheated on. When Stacey found out that her longtime partner had been unfaithful, her immediate reaction was to question what she had done to deserve it. Her partner had so effectively infiltrated her thinking that she blamed herself, even when confronted with evidence. She remembers reflecting in the moment she found out, "I let him push my boundaries so much, and he's still [cheating]."

Stacey chose to call her partner to confront him. Looking back, she recognizes she did this because the phone felt much safer than confronting someone face-to-face who was already hurting her behind closed doors. Her choice makes a lot of sense, and survivors in abusive relationships often choose nontraditional means of resisting our abusers in order to prioritize safety.

Looking back, Stacey realizes it was easier to explain a breakup caused by infidelity—everybody would support her for leaving in that case—rather than to break her silence about the abuse, which would lead to more complicated conversations. Cheating was much easier to talk about openly. We, as a culture, haven't yet developed the language to describe why she stayed, and like many survivors, she felt accountable for staying, like she needed to explain those choices in order to ask for help in leaving.

Instead of apologizing or trying to salvage the relationship, her partner told Stacey the relationship was done. They were over. While they were still on the phone, Stacey's car crashed. She was in a serious accident. Her car was totaled and she suffered both a neck and traumatic brain injury. She had frontal lobe damage and wasn't able to cognitively function. Stacey's would-be ex used her injury to reposition himself back into her life. Stacey sees now that her abusive partner took advantage of her injury and disability, reversing the breakup and becoming involved in her life while she recovered. In her cognitively impaired state, she wasn't able to keep him away.

Going back to a partner she had technically broken up with looks "bad" from an outsider's perspective. In Stacey's extreme circumstance, being physically disabled might lessen that shame and judgment—she couldn't move even if she wanted to. But when it comes to sexual violence, and especially sustained relationships, somehow, all survivors seem to come off looking "bad." It isn't complicated, really. We hold sexual assault survivors up to impossible standards so that we don't have to face reality: that sexual assault is pervasive, out of the victim's control, and entrenched in our culture.

Many people believe the narrative of the "perfect" victim: the victim who fights back physically and verbally throughout the entire assault. The victim who immediately flees the scene. The victim who doesn't turn around, doesn't look back, hoping to never see the perpetrator again or sure that this person will be punished. This perfect victim is a myth.

Some of our judgment of victims is based on a lack of understanding about how people respond when subjected to sexual violence. Fight or flight is our popular understanding of the basic human response to danger. However, research suggests two other responses: freeze or appease. Freeze often entails becoming rigid and silent during an assault. Post-assault, freeze often involves denial or becoming stuck in the moment of the attack, on high alert. Appease, also called tend and befriend, may explain why victims sometimes continue a relationship with a perpetrator. Rather than remove oneself from a dangerous situation, the desire for social support and affiliation with another person may be strong enough that a victim may turn to the only person they feel close to—the perpetrator. The tend and befriend response is particularly prevalent among women.[1]

While Stacey returned to work and took steps toward recovery, she was living in a haze for a year. In public, her partner looked supportive, helping her get around and manage her injuries. But behind closed doors, not only was he still abusive, but he used her injuries to further control her. She had three herniated discs from the accident, and her neck was misshapen while she recovered. Her partner would grab her by the neck and move her around the apartment so that she was in so much pain that she was forced to comply. Resisting his grip hurt more, and she felt trapped. He made fun of her as she struggled.

After damage to her frontal lobe, Stacey was operating in a fog. But the cheating she'd learned about just before the accident was still on her mind. One day eight months after the accident, while her partner was out, she picked up his tablet and entered the password. Stacey reflects that it was one of her first moments of clear thinking post-car accident. It only took a couple of taps to figure out that while she was recovering from serious injuries—and while he was manipulating her into staying with him so he could abuse her—he had continued to cheat on her. In a fury, Stacey gathered up all of the stuff she kept at his apartment, packed her cat in a travel carrier, and drove to the apartment she still rented, though she didn't live there anymore.

Stacey, like many survivors of domestic violence, had an intuitive understanding that leaving would be dangerous. She had also studied and worked in this area for years. But she knew she had to finish what she had set out to do almost a year earlier: leave him. This time, she did two things differently, which were key to her safety. First, she let a friend know she was in danger because she was leaving her partner. Then she allowed that friend to help her leave. She accepted her offer to stay with her because she knew that would be safer than the apartment she knew he would go looking for her at.

Telling a friend we don't feel safe, whether in a relationship or in another context, is scary. We don't know what the friend's reaction will be, and there's a chance they might respond with judgment or even withdraw, unwilling or unable to handle the situation. To navigate this challenge, it's important to stay centered in your own experience. What would you feel comfortable with this friend knowing, even if they don't react well? What do you need from a friend? A place to stay? Assistance accessing resources to help you leave safely? Maybe you just need someone to listen so you can say what's happening to you out loud. If you can articulate not only what's happening but also your needs, you're setting yourself up for a better reaction, giving the other person the opportunity to give you exactly what you need. And if they don't respond in a helpful way, you can ask another friend for help, or not—it's up to you.

One of my survivor friends, a straight woman, found support in online forums for sexual assault survivors, where she could post and reply freely about sexual issues behind an anonymous username. She also took steps to set up a support system in real life. After moving around a lot throughout her life, she knew she needed more of a home base to rely on, and she reconnected with childhood friends who she knew would be there for her for the long run. Many other survivors found support in a group of understanding friends, too. Survivors like Alexis, a straight woman, turned to activism to gain a community. Now, her social circle includes many anti-sexual violence advocates, who have the training to talk to her about her sexual issues in an informed, compassionate way. While some survivors felt that talking about sexual issues related to trauma was too uncomfortable a topic to broach with family, others have close relationships with relatives who they can turn to for support.

If you are the friend of a survivor who comes to you for help, always try to center the survivor's needs, not your own experience of learning about what happened to them. Ask what they need and offer to help however you can. If you have a strong reaction to what the survivor tells you, express your emotions in a supportive way, by validating their experience and listening actively, not as an attempt to make yourself feel better, without considering how that affects the survivor.

Sometimes, we don't have friends who can help us—or we don't have access to them, stuck in a cycle of violence. In that case, to get to safety we might need to ask for outside support. Survivors I spoke to describe how helpful a hotline, like the National Domestic Violence Hotline, or even chatting with a representative from a local domestic violence organization online can be. Not only are these resources helpful in figuring out how to get more help, but they can also prove reassuring for people who are otherwise isolated from typical sources of validation, like friends or family. The people on the other end of the line can help you figure out what aspects of your experience should not be tolerated or are dangerous so you don't have to figure it out alone.

There's a lot of pressure to have a clean break when ending a relationship, but when leaving domestic violence relationships, the highest priority has to be safety—no matter how that looks on the outside. If you take away the fact that the relationship was deeply abusive, Stacey's breakup looks messy to outsiders. After she'd recovered enough from her accident to leave him, she didn't have an official breakup conversation with her abuser. She still texted him occasionally but lived apart from him and let the relationship deteriorate. This space gave Stacey the room to mentally begin to move on in a safer environment, until she was ready to break up with him officially. While slowly leaving a serious partner may be frowned upon, this only applies to non-abusive relationships. A survivor should do whatever they need to in order to leave safely and shouldn't be shamed for it. In these cases, it's important to think of the (ex-) partner as a perpetrator of violence and the survivor as somebody using every tool in their toolbox to get away.

While sources of support like a domestic violence hotline can help you take early steps toward safety, they aren't a replacement for actually leaving an abusive context. Survivors I spoke to confirmed time and again that staying with an abuser is antithetical to healing.

Of all the survivors I spoke to, those still involved with their assailants were, in many ways, the most confused. They see their assaults as an imbalance of power but don't necessarily see the perpetrators as threats, despite the fact that statistically, perpetrators sexually assault repeatedly. It's not always a one-time instance, as much as victims hope. The survivors I spoke to who were still involved with their attackers often took longer to recognize their assaults as violations and to begin to approach sex in a more embodied, healthy way—and that healthy reclamation universally only happened after they actually left the abusive partner.

When I first interviewed Mia, a bisexual woman, she disclosed that not only had she been assaulted in college, but she'd experienced an additional assault just a few months before we spoke. This time, it was at the hands of a new partner. At that time, Mia was still in a sexual relationship with the man who raped her years before. She felt that sleeping with the perpetrator seemed like a way of taking her power back. She was confused about whether to stop trusting this man completely—hadn't it only been one time? She'd known this man since college; at least he was a known quantity. She told him what he did was wrong. He gave a half-hearted apology. Doesn't an apology count for anything? she wondered. She kept dating him. Within the confines of rape culture, Mia's perspective isn't entirely unreasonable. How often are victims of violence, especially women, told that it could be so much worse? Mia perceived the completely unknown partner as scarier than the known one, even in the face of evidence to the contrary.

Mia explained to me how she'd spent decades absorbing the message that as a Black woman, she should be able to grit her teeth through whatever life threw at her. Even after a rape, she should be able to pick herself up, dust herself off, and move forward as if nothing had happened. In this case, that meant trying to move past the rape and preserve the relationship with her attacker. Mia's mother, who knew about the assault, begged Mia to leave him. But Mia was sure that as a white woman, her mother couldn't understand the pressures she felt as a Black woman. The standards for their reactions felt so different, split along racial lines. Mia ignored her mother's advice.

Mia told me, repeatedly, that she felt like she could have prevented it. She had been assaulted before. How could this have happened again? It must be something about her—not him. Mia made jokes at her own expense, yet the pain of her horrible situation, the blunt facts of it, made cracks in the facade she was trying to keep up—a facade she seemed desperate to uphold.

At the time of our first conversation, Mia still slept with the man who attacked her, but she had other male sexual partners as well. At some point after, Mia, who identifies as bisexual, decided to drop men and exclusively seek out relationships with women. Though the fear and resistance she felt toward men was absent from her relationships with women, something was still off about sex. She kept being drawn back toward sex with men, particularly sex with her assailant. It felt like a battle she was determined to win. Over and over again, she tried to gain back what she'd lost, to reach back and protect herself from him, but it didn't matter how many times she tried to have healthy sex with him; she could not escape the fact that he was her rapist. It's impossible to give consent retroactively, and Mia couldn't quite come to terms with that fact.

Being trapped in a relationship with an abuser means being trapped in the position of victim, like a song stuck on loop. Some survivors, seeking to silence that awful sound, try to assert power in a shattered relationship. They hope to regain a sense of control over the past and present—but it's impossible, and unsafe. Victimization is a pattern that can only be broken by removing oneself from the position of being harmed. We are victims of crimes, but the healing process necessarily moves us into a new identity, a new framework: survivors. It is within this adopted armor that we begin to heal.

I spoke to Mia a year after our first interview. She was only just then emerging from the relationship with her perpetrator. The true nature of her relationship had recently become clearer to her. Ultimately, it wasn't any conversation she had with somebody who loved her, or a big realization about how he had treated her, that got her to leave. One night, after seeing him after a party, she realized that while she had once thought highly of him as a person—"he was the most interesting person in the world in college"—she now saw that he had no ambition, that he hadn't grown since they met, and that he was boring. She stopped responding to his texts, and that was that. In the end, Mia stopped her relationship with him not because he was a threat, but because he wasn't a viable partner. While this may sound like poor decision-making, any decision to leave a violent partner is a good one and should be affirmed.

Unfortunately, had she gotten out sooner, she would likely have carried less of a psychic burden—traumatic stress compounded by an extended period of heightened danger. She felt weighed down as she struggled to move forward, making her suffer from poor mental health and relationship issues. But Mia's outlook ultimately changed for the better. When she and I last spoke, she shared that her entire perspective evolved after she finally stopped sleeping with the first rapist.

Today, Mia expresses the desire to share her story with her nieces—when they're older—to explain the importance of bodily autonomy. At first, she was hesitant to own how bad it was out loud, since she believed her rape could have been worse; it could have been more violent than what she experienced. Mia shared that our conversation made her reconsider how she would describe the rape. She realized that if it happened to somebody else, she would never discount it, "violent" or not, so she shouldn't discount her own experience. Whether or not it was violent or physically damaging seemed less important to her the longer she talked about it. That mental flexibility, that perspective shift, was something only available to her because she left her partner.

Additional perspective shifts may have to emerge to move forward from an abusive relationship or prolonged assaults. The baseline understanding of how healthy sexual encounters work—that you can say no at any time—is a positive outlook that shatters when faced with mounting evidence that the world doesn't actually work like that. The just world belief, or a balanced worldview, that takes good for good and bad for bad, can be a challenging perspective to hold for survivors. To move forward from assault, we have to learn to assert our boundaries, whether or not they were respected in the past.

There are other significant impacts of staying in a threatening situation. Many experts recommend taking a "sex vacation" after an assault, a period to give your body—and expectations about your body—a break. This is impossible in a relationship with an abuser because of a power dynamic where the victim is under the abuser's control—or at least, it feels that way. It's possible that following an assault, a victim could have consensual sex with the perpetrator, at least according to the legal definition of consent. That sex might even appear healthy. However, that sex is happening between people with a very skewed power dynamic. But sex problems don't necessarily show up right away. Even if an assault in the relationship doesn't seem to have an effect on a survivor's sex life, it's very possible it will make itself known later on. Some survivors say that sleeping with their perpetrators is a form of self-hatred or self-destructiveness. And if the survivor's abusive relationship is with their first-ever partner, it can be doubly confusing, because they don't have an existing experience to compare the abuse to.

When Libby, a pansexual woman, met her first boyfriend, she was a junior in high school. Few people at her small private school were dating, and students who wanted to try out romance often turned to their peers at other schools. Libby ended up looking elsewhere, too, but the boyfriend she found wasn't from another high school—he wasn't in school at all. Ten years older than she was, this man appealed to Libby. Dating an older guy made her feel mature, powerful, and a step above her friends who were dating boys the same age as her.

Libby had never had sex when she met her boyfriend, and had no real idea of what sex was or how it might feel to her. She could not conceptualize, let alone enact, sexual agency given the imbalance of power caused by their age difference. She wasn't old enough to consent. She believed he knew better, so when he wanted to have sex, she acquiesced. Looking back, she sees it as clear-cut statutory rape in an inherently abusive relationship.

At the time, though, Libby didn't see it that way. "For women, there's a sense that our bodies and sex don't belong to us to begin with," Libby said. For her, rape was confirmation of an existing, culturally enforced belief about how sex worked.

Libby stayed in that relationship for years. Without previous dating or sexual experience, Libby believed what was happening was normal. Raped many times by her boyfriend, she came to believe that sex was about her partner's control, her partner's orgasm, fulfilling somebody else's needs. She developed ideas about sex that enabled her to continue to see their relationship as healthy, even as—over the course of months, then years—she began to realize it wasn't. As in Libby's case, assault may feel more like coercion than force, which some victims find easier to ignore or deny. Nobody wants to believe something horrible happened to them, let alone that something horrible is continuing to happen. And if the assailant was somebody the victim trusted, even loved, somebody with whom they continue to build a relationship afterward, it's easy for the victim to start to question their experience of the event. *Maybe they didn't hear me. Maybe they thought I was playing hard to get. Maybe I didn't push them off firmly enough for them to know I was serious.*

Years after the initial assault, Libby's abusive relationship ended. Like Stacey, like Mia, her breakup wasn't explicitly caused by the assaults, or any major reckoning with her abuser. The couple, so different in age, drifted apart. Libby went away to college, and like so many other freshmen surrounded by new, friendly faces and the opportunity to start again, she shed her hometown boyfriend. As years passed and she gained distance from her high school relationship abuse, Libby started to process more clearly the violation she'd experienced. Being robbed of something before she clearly knew what it was, and then staying in a relationship in which that was the norm, was destabilizing to her growth and sexual self-expression for almost a decade. Instead of being the jumping-off point to exploring her sexuality, as she had hoped back in high school, the relationship proved to be destructive.

Trauma can damage a person's idea of who they are, their self-conception, and make them redefine themselves to fit the context in which they were assaulted. Libby managed to reclaim her sense of self in college and after, but remains wary of trusting any sexual partner too soon. She says that now she prefers to wait longer to choose to have sex with a new partner, believing it makes sex better. This belief was reinforced by her experience of the opposite: of not having a choice at all.

When survivors continue relationships where abuse is being perpetrated, we may be seeking stability—but we're doing it with the people who destabilize us most, and it will never work. The stakes are high for leaving. And for some, leaving isn't such a clear decision. As Jennifer put it, safety isn't normalized in sexual relationships, especially for women. In order for victims to recognize that what's happening is wrong, the standards for how we should be treated need to be clearer, and higher. Ignacio G. Rivera, a queer trans nonbinary survivor, put it bluntly: "Consent is the low bar." We need a clearer vision for what sex and relationships can look like outside the domain of rape culture.

For many, a feeling of safety can first be located in our bodies: How does your body feel in this environment around this person? A friend once described to me something experts have suggested: You need your brain, your heart, and your body to all say yes to sex. If one of those things is missing, my friend pauses to rethink the encounter. If it's impossible to maintain a baseline physical safety in a relationship, it likely is not a space in which sexual healing can take place. You can't take healthy risks and grow if you are actually in danger. Post-traumatic growth is only possible from a position of safety and security.

When survivors do get out of these relationships, what's next? How can we set ourselves up to move forward safely? Approaching sexual healing, even reading about it, can be a distressing experience, bringing up emotions and questions that are difficult to face on our own.

So how do we find support? Some survivors seek support through college campus rape centers or religious organizations we're a part of. Sometimes, though, we experience abuse inside these communities and have to leave these comfortable environments. Gabby Gomez, a bisexual woman, described how getting psychological support was harder outside of the infrastructure of a college campus. Upon graduating, all of the support she had relied on evaporated. How was she supposed to navigate being a sexual assault survivor and the manager of a company? Where was she supposed to find quality mental health services? Who was available to talk to about the sexual issues she faced, besides the people she was sleeping with? It took years of trial and error to regain the sense of support she'd had in college.

Much of the time, recovering a sex life after sexual assault may feel like running away from fear. And if you are trapped in an unsafe situation, getting away is a crucial first step. But we can begin to reframe recovery, looking not only at the past, but forward, into the future. Instead of escaping pain, it can be about goals: What do you want your sex life to look like moving forward? This future-oriented healing means a partner can help you meet these goals. Instead of seeking to prevent things that scare you, sexual assault survivors can seek out things they want, even find sexual role models. In the absence of threat, what kind of sexual identity do each of us want to cultivate?

Having a supportive partner—and not an abusive one—can help support sexual healing. And many survivors I spoke to agree that choosing a safe partner is a personal and difficult process, particular to our past and present needs. But missing from these conversations is an acknowledgment that no matter how hard you try to choose somebody who is safe, anybody can end up in a relationship with somebody who has hurt, or is hurting, them. It's impossible to know for sure that somebody will never hurt you, and "getting it wrong" is never your fault. You can't control what other people say or do to you.

So, how can we center our sex and relationships around safety? You can never be 100 percent certain the person or environment you've chosen will be safe for you forever. But you can make the decision that if something becomes unsafe, uncomfortable, or simply unwanted, you can leave. In the past, I've given the advice, "Before making any choices about the future, your body needs to calm down." It's impossible to move toward what you really want, in sex, relationships, or life at all, if you have your back against a wall, gun to your head, or are backed into a corner—sometimes literally. That kind of stress impacts your ability to think clearly and make a solid plan to get out. In order to retreat into safety, focusing on skills that will help you feel physically safer—from taking time for yourself to spending a weekend away visiting family—can help clear your head. And there's no point in trying to repair a sex life with somebody who is a constant source of stress or trauma. First, safety must be established. No matter how complicated it is to extricate yourself from a threat—you can always leave.

It's not guaranteed that leaving her partner immediately after the first time he assaulted her would have prevented the next few years of traumatic stress Stacey endured. But leaving likely would have helped. Research shows that the number one determining factor for how quickly and effectively sexual assault survivors recover is whether or not they have a supportive partner. In my interviews, I've found that the reverse can be true too. If, instead of a nurturing, understanding partner, a survivor is partnered with the perpetrator, it's even harder to move on than for a survivor who is single. A loved one's bad reaction—almost a guarantee if that loved one is the perpetrator—can often erode the victim's trust even beyond the traumatic event itself. Staying in a relationship with an abuser may result in further instances of assault too. Prolonged trauma—multiple instances of violence over a long period of time—can lead to complex post-traumatic stress disorder (C-PTSD).

This compounds the difficulty of healing and regaining a sex life. Staying in a relationship with the perpetrator can intensify traumatic stress, prevent survivors from accessing social support, and inflict an additional layer of psychic pain. But it can also be approached like a simple math equation. Leaving sooner shifts the balance of time: less time in pain, more time to heal.

Some C-PTSD symptoms fall outside the range of typical PTSD symptoms and speak more toward how trauma becomes embedded in our personality and how we relate to others.[2] When trauma is built into how we approach relationships, we may struggle more to recenter ourselves and enter relationships from our own perspective. While leaving an abusive relationship may be helpful in preventing C-PTSD, in a way we are all exposed to the trauma of rape culture on a regular basis, and the aggregate of those experiences may change our behavior just as ongoing abuse affects our later relationships. Regardless of the underlying threat causing distress, it's key to our survival moving forward to recognize how sexual assault affects us.

Ramona recently had a moment with her boyfriend that called into question the definition of a "safe person." They were hooking up but had a longstanding understanding that they wouldn't have intercourse most of the time, and definitely not without talking first. Suddenly, Ramona thought he was starting to have intercourse with her. She felt startled and began to cry. For several minutes, she sobbed. She didn't understand why she was so upset, because she knew he wouldn't actually initiate intercourse without her consent. In the moment, he reaffirmed that he would never cross a defined boundary. She completely believed him, and it made her wonder how she could end up with the fear response she did if she trusted him as a person. She realized that sometimes, trauma rears its head even when she's with someone who feels genuinely, completely safe. It was a loaded moment, and her response wasn't a reflection of his safety as a partner. Sometimes the two aren't related, and it's helpful to keep a flexible idea of what makes us feel safe versus what keeps us actually safe.

Survivors are experts in our own experiences, our own bodies, and our own safety. When Leanna Lee, a straight woman, thinks of a safe person, she thinks of words like reliable, dependable, and respectful.

But she recognizes that she sees those same terms thrown around as negatives when it comes to dating—they can mean "boring." Leanna still asserts that these qualities "are the core tenets of a healthy relationship." For her in particular, it's important that a "safe" person be comfortable and secure enough in themselves to take criticism, or at least not get fazed if she has a different opinion or concern about the relationship or their sex life. She wants a partner to be "both comfortable within themselves and open to changing so that they're able to make adjustments without losing their sense of identity," Leanna explains. For example, Leanna's husband has always been more physically affectionate than her, but he tones it down in their relationship because it bothers her. He doesn't change who he is, and at the same time doing less PDA doesn't threaten his sense of self. "It's really hard to be in a relationship with someone who resents any changes, any boundaries that you have, because they think it'll change them, or because they want to control you in any way," Leanna says. She never wants to compromise on her hard boundaries but believes a relationship won't work if either party feels those boundaries endanger their sense of who they are or who their partner is.

As important as it is to feel your fear so you can recognize it and then set your boundaries to protect yourself, there are circumstances when you are not in a safe place to feel your feelings. Somatics is a type of bodywork that helps you focus on your own physical and personal experience. Lexi, a somatic wellness coach, remembers hearing something powerful in training: "containment is fine." She learned that at times it's healthy to hold emotions in because it's not always safe to feel your feelings. For example, when Lexi got triggered at work when men walked up behind her in the hallway, that wasn't a safe place to feel her feelings, process what happened, and move through it. "You can put that in a little box and put it down," Lexi explains. But containment is only temporary. Long-term, containment isn't healthy. What you put in that box can start to fester and grow without you even noticing and become much bigger than it was to begin with. But setting aside processing something for three hours, or a day, or a week, to be able to then take it out in a safe space and slowly start to process it in a safe container has healing potential beyond what being able to immediately process something would necessarily offer.

Clients will now come to Lexi in her somatics practice, unboxing triggered moments from the past week so they can feel them in a session with her. Lexi first asks her clients how it feels in their body to acknowledge that there is a box to look at. If acknowledging that feels overwhelming, they stay at the level of acknowledging that there is something there that feels really big. Until they become grounded in that, they won't move forward. The next question might be, how does reaching toward the box and opening it feel? If you're disconnected from the moment where the trigger happened, you get to notice more closely than if you were able to feel it at the time you got activated. She might ask her client which parts feel more overwhelming and which parts are actually less triggering than they might have expected from that surface level. This process of containment can be helpful to survivors who are dealing with the fallout of sexual trauma, but not living in an environment they feel completely safe in. It's not always healthy to immediately feel our feelings, and setting aside our reaction for a later time may allow us to process them more openly and fully. Plus, if you have other people whose reactions to your processing are necessary to consider, like your kids or your boss, learning to contain your initial reaction and save it for later is a survival skill.

The ability to contain those unsafe feelings only helps if you have a safe space in which to check in with yourself. Leaving unsafe relationships and minimizing threats from other sources is a necessary precursor to reaching those safe spaces. Leaving somebody who is a threat may be scary, but on the other side, you'll find something beyond just safety. You'll find yourself.

CHAPTER 2

Check In with Yourself

A S A CHILD, I experienced sexual assault by a female peer. At that young age, I did not have the words to explain what happened, nor did I have the words to describe my sexuality and my confusion over it. Growing up, I was attracted to girls my age and, later, women, but felt stuck, unable to act on my feelings, because the gender identity of my abuser matched the gender of some of the people I felt attracted to. Any therapy I did as a child completely glossed over the sexual aspects of those assaults, and growth as a sexual human being was never the focus. My school sex ed was mostly about anatomy. Even as a young adult, for a long time, I avoided publicly identifying as bisexual or dating women.

In college, my friend introduced me to a student in her program. Her name was Sarah, and I was mesmerized. She had soft, dark brown hair that swirled as she danced around my room. We were both in college for creative majors and going through recent trauma. It felt like we would never run out of things to talk about, and we easily built emotional intimacy. I loved how she ran her fingers through my hair and across my collarbone. I loved staying up all night talking, lying together in our dorm beds, ignoring roommates and homework. But I held back, physically. I didn't want to disrupt the image I had of myself, someone who could simply choose to date only men and avoid having to deal with a broader sexuality, as well as an entire area of post-trauma sexual healing altogether. Sarah was the first woman I even considered going beyond just kissing, though I hesitated around oral sex. It felt too tied up in trauma—with anybody, not just women.

Years later, when a new friend suggested that if I was hesitant about receiving oral, I wasn't really bi, I felt all the old shame around being told I was faking a sexuality that I actually have, just because of my trauma's impact on my sexual preferences. Sexual self-definition is important for everybody; it allows us to claim bodily autonomy, desire, and determine what kind of partner or relationship we want. But for survivors, sexual identity is complicated not only by our pasts, but also by what society expects of us.

Back in college, I was unaware of all of this. I just knew that I had romantic feelings about Sarah and was unsure what to make of them. One night I approached my roommates, my closest friends at the time. I'd told them about kissing girls I liked, but never labeled myself as bisexual. So I simply said, "I think I like Sarah."

My roommates responded as a chorus:

"But you're straight."

"So you're just leading her on."

"You're probably going to hurt her feelings."

"You're just her friend."

"You're straight."

Struggling to articulate the real reason I felt hesitant to hook up with her—my unaddressed trauma history and its impact on dating in general, but also women specifically—I chose their narrative: that I was straight. I rebuffed Sarah the next chance I got, and disappeared from her life. I was crushed to learn Sarah left our school a few months later, that everything I'd hoped to find with her was now a continent away.

For years, I stuck to my roommates' narrative. Eventually I emerged from my shell and sought out women I was interested in. I found more supportive communities. I adopted the label "bi" as if it were easy, as if it had always been easy. Avoiding pursuing a relationship with Sarah remained one of my biggest sexual regrets for a long time. I think if I had had somebody to talk with about the real reason I hesitated—her gender and the gender of my childhood assailant—I might not have hesitated at all. If I'd centered my own experiences, of trust, sexuality, the relationship, instead of focusing on others' experiences and perspectives, I could have made choices for myself—a healing act in itself. My sexual healing was never going to be anybody else's priority, and I learned the hard way that I had to make it mine.

It's easy to get caught up in other people's perspectives about our sex lives post-assault. Partners, friends, doctors may all envision something different for us than we would choose. Even researchers and experts boil survivors down into statistics, numbers. But at the end of the day, the only perspective that really matters is your own. None of us are "just a number"—we're individuals with singular lives. Owning what you want, need, and don't want is an internal process you have to engage in not just before you have sex for the first time after assault, but in an ongoing way, built into your sex life moving forward.

It's becoming common to check in with your partner during sex, but after speaking with dozens of sexual assault survivors, I wholeheartedly recommend redistributing some of that attention to checking in with yourself. This means before, during, and after sex. What influences your current perspective on sex and relationships? What examples are you looking to for what a healthy sex life looks like? What toxic aspects of your sex education or reaction to trauma are holding you back? The first step to growth is awareness. In addition to checking in with yourself mentally, self-awareness also relates to the body, including being aware of your own physical reactions to situations, people, and changes in your environment.

Many survivors feel like PTSD is embedded in our lives, impossible to unpick from other influences. Nearly a decade after her assault, Leanna still rarely goes out after dark. She tells me she is afraid of her own shadow, of walking alone, or of having somebody creep up behind her at night. That restriction all but wipes out her social life after sundown, especially in the winter. Some therapists might call her decision to abide by that limitation avoidance, but in the greater hierarchy of all her triggers, this is fairly minor. When a trigger or an impact of trauma has persisted for a very long time, Leanna thinks it becomes more part of her than part of her illness. "I don't think there really is a way of reversing them," Leanna says of her most ingrained triggers. Every time I spoke to Leanna, I found her honesty around what she thinks her baseline looks like refreshing. So often, survivors are told to constantly strive to be free from the impact of trauma. But that can make us feel worse in the moment, when we're still struggling. It's normal to have significant triggers after sexual assault, and it's normal for sexual assault to impact your sex life—even if you expect those things to get easier in the future. It's okay to be struggling right now.

Leanna brings up a difficult reality that many survivors face: No matter how much we work on PTSD symptoms or trauma fallout, often, trauma persists. For me, this looks like an aversion to having my wrists touched, even lightly or nonsexually. I have done exposure therapy on the topic, but I have also had later harassment and assaults reinforce the idea that being touched on the wrists is dangerous. When we are living in circumstances that reinforce our avoidance, it can be hard to break out of that avoidance.

Avoidance can also be a means of trying to preserve stability. If, after an assault, a survivor regains a sense of safety but hasn't yet coped with certain triggers, they may opt to stay within that created sense of security and reassurance for as long as possible. We may just need more time before diving into therapy, or sex, or a relationship. Avoiding dating may have more to do with avoiding the negative feelings that come with it (trauma-related or otherwise) than the process of dating itself, especially if you're only just starting to feel better.

When the pandemic shut down her gym, Lexi turned to running. Because of the widespread shutdown, a lot more people joined her running route. Lexi quickly noticed that anytime a man ran up behind her and she couldn't see him, her energy "tightened." So, she turned to a somatics coach.

Lexi tells me that somatics is a type of bodywork that emphasizes how you perceive your own physical and personal experience. She had such personal success doing bodywork with her own coach that she felt compelled to pursue a career around somatics herself. Together with her coach, she started body scanning, or spending time noticing physical sensations from across her body, piece by piece. Through this noticing-based practice, Lexi started rebuilding and facilitating safety in her body. Lexi's coach asked her to start by questioning her experience: When are the moments you feel a lack of trust in your body? By looking at her present relationship with her own body, and not focusing on past traumatic moments where somebody else was in control, Lexi began to understand her triggers and the contexts where her nervous system response was more elevated, even if she wasn't having a full flashback or panic attack. When she practiced boundaries with her somatics coach, she paid attention to what creating and enforcing those boundaries felt like within her body, not just how she thought about them in her head. Her coach helped her slow way down, helping Lexi build more of an awareness of the sensations coursing through her, good or bad. Lexi learned what many survivors learn: Sometimes triggers or the panic reactions that come with them have more to do with pacing than the specific issue at hand. Most triggers can be tackled in bite-size chunks. It was only after Lexi spent time sitting with those sensations, checking in with her physical response to stimuli, that she was able to fully communicate about them with others. Her ability to communicate was honed after much self-education, going back and relearning the basics of sex and relationships for herself.

I asked every survivor I spoke to for this book to describe their sex education, whether formal or informal. The answers ranged widely, from comprehensive sexuality education from the Unitarian Church to homeschooled abstinence-only education to heteronormative methods that simply do not apply to real life, and beyond. In these discussions we took apart how early experiences of sexuality and contextual knowledge about sex and relationships influenced our own responses to trauma, especially when it comes to sex. Some people found their early education useful, but many found it damaging, and had to unlearn those early messages in order to heal from later trauma. Ultimately, survivors found that taking on the project of "sex educating" ourselves after trauma can be useful moving forward, no matter our sex education background—or sexual experience prior to assault. Learning about our sexual selves and the world of sex will only make our sex lives better.

Campus administrations hire Stacey to talk about sexual assault through the lens of Title IX, the federal law that aims to protect students from discrimination on the basis of sex. This is a very narrow legal lens to explore something as vast as the intersection of sexuality and violence. Stacey has been doing this work since before she experienced sexual assault herself. When she gives presentations about consent as part of Title IX programs, she uses humor and a balance of talking about sexuality and trauma to educate young people about sex, and ultimately impact the future of sexuality and sexual violence prevention.

Before Stacey taught about sex professionally, she had very little sex education. As a little kid, she learned to keep her hands to herself, but then it was radio silence for years—going to Catholic school didn't help. She only learned about sex from porn or movies, and looking back, Stacey says she's horrified about how those images got translated in her mind, particularly the idea that what she was seeing was how sex actually worked: somebody just "does stuff to you." She now sees how porn failed her. "It doesn't teach people how to be sexually assertive while still respecting someone else's sexual agency," she points out, referencing that in porn, consent conversations are very often literally behind the scenes.

Stacey's first exposure to formal sex education was as a first-year student in college. She watched somebody roll a condom onto a dildo. "I was shook to my core," Stacey remembers. Her early life naivete compelled her to want to educate people. At the same time, she developed close friendships with fellow female students who were very secure in their femininity, their sexuality, and their reproductive rights—many worked at Planned Parenthood. Conversations around sex came up naturally, and Stacey feels most of her real, meaningful sex ed came from those college friends.

As a sexuality student, one of the first things Stacey had to go through was a Sexual Attitudes Reassessment (SAR). She describes it as intentional, intense exposure to sexually explicit material (or, in her words, "basically watching porn for two days"), with a group of fellow students. Over the course of the multiday experience, the group stopped to debrief a few times. She wishes that everybody, not just sexuality educators, could have this experience, because it really opened her eyes. She had to ask herself why certain things made her feel aroused that she had never previously associated with sex—some of it even seemed gross at the same time. *What is happening here?* Stacey asked herself. *Why am I having such a strong disgust reaction to this?* She broke down a lot of internalized messages through the process. Today, she helps run SARs and facilitates the debriefs.

In the early years of Stacey's career, she was the victim in an abusive relationship. She had already begun working as a sexual health educator and was an advocate for sexual assault survivors—while experiencing assault herself. She put others' needs before her own. After she got out of that relationship, she decided to go back to school again so she would be more qualified to educate people. As she learned more about sexuality as well as abuse, Stacey began to ask herself how she could apply what she was learning to her own life. Her education, originally intended to help her help others, ended up helping her on her own healing path.

Stacey didn't plan to go to school to heal herself. She started down this path just absorbing everything around her. "There's so much value in people being able to learn about sexuality in a nonjudgmental way," Stacey says. You get to ask what you're learning means for you. In her case, she would then navigate the space as an individual and as a professional. She wishes more people had the space to reassess their sexuality after trauma and sees formal sexuality education as one arena that feels safe enough to do it.

For Ignacio, the trans nonbinary survivor, it took getting older and gaining access to more educational materials that allowed them to claim the labels and narratives that proved most useful to them. Today, Ignacio is a cultural sociologist with experience in sexual trauma and healing for marginalized populations. Now they can educate others, but back when they were a kid, they experienced a huge education deficit. Ignacio, age fifty-two when we spoke, recalls going to the young adult section of the library, or even the adult section, as a kid, searching for stories about sexual abuse, for books that reflected back Ignacio's lived experience. "That shifted things for me," Ignacio says, nodding. Before finding those stories, Ignacio remembers having crushes on people and passing notes to them, or acting out scenes they'd watched on TV with people they thought they could go out with. They were completely ignoring their intuition at that point—about their identity and attraction—and nothing felt right. Some messaging Ignacio received was destructive, like the idea that boys pull girls' hair to show they like them. Ignacio points out that plants a seed of domestic violence, and the kind of thinking that might cause a grown woman to hesitate before leaving a man that's hurting her.

Ignacio still felt a disconnect between acknowledging sexual violation and trauma, and healing sex and sexuality. Ignacio feels that disconnect is damaging and slows the process of repair. When we don't maintain that connection between trauma and sex, we're not being vulnerable enough to authentically share with empathy and compassion. So much has been "derailed from the harm that was done."

Despite all of their reading and independent research, Ignacio was inundated with negative messaging related to healing: "It was just like, stay away from sex. Don't even talk about sex. It's all about power and control, power and control, power and control." There were no models of healthy sexuality that took into account trauma histories or the way trauma impacts sex. While Ignacio didn't have sex ed in the traditional classroom sense, they recognize how much their mother influenced their understanding of the impact of trauma on sex. If Ignacio asked her a question about something sexual, they were shut down out of fear of sex or pregnancy. When Ignacio tried to point out the abuse they were suffering at the hands of their sister, Ignacio's mom was completely ignorant to the idea that any kind of abuse even could be happening, believing in the still-popular binary that men are rapists and women are victims, and that we shouldn't talk about abuse inside a family. This gaslighting, even if unintentional, proved immensely damaging to Ignacio's healing and delayed their sexual development long after the assaults were over.

Although Ignacio can see that their mother was doing her best, now that they're a parent and grandparent themself, it looks different. Ignacio sees this updated perspective as essential to handling child sexual abuse, because children have no power at the time they are abused. It's really the adults that raise and nurture them that have the tools to create a culture where kids aren't harmed, and they can recognize what is right and wrong. As adults, we get to the place "where we're really unraveling what happened to us," Ignacio says, pointing out that "many people never get there." So many of us are just struggling to survive day-to-day, and accessing the resources necessary to heal sexually after sexual assault is not our present reality. Many of us follow made-up cultural rules in relationships, without being in touch with our intuition. Our day-to-day lives may not offer much room for emotional growth.

Several survivors of childhood sexual abuse pointed out that they didn't have any grounding in sexuality before they were assaulted. All the healing work they did, afterward, was future-oriented; there was nothing to reclaim from their past. Survivors who experienced sexual assault as a child may not have a sexual self-definition to return to, and may spend adolescence searching for validation of their trauma. Sexuality, for them, evolves after abuse. Ignacio recalls being "utterly confused about how to actually have a relationship and connect with people outside of what society tells you," on an intimate and individual level. They remember following what felt like a script for how they're supposed to flirt or be sexual with anybody, even as a little kid. At the same time, Ignacio received next to no education about sexual assault, and wasn't even sure what to call the sexual abuse they endured.

Alisa, a straight woman, was sexually abused as a child, like Ignacio. As she tried to claim her own sexual agency as an adolescent and young adult, she felt uncomfortable with an onslaught of information from health-care professionals pathologizing her post-trauma sexual experiences. Learning about the topic only from professionals made her feel "like I was some traumatized lab rat talking about the hypersexuality of girl survivors." Whichever direction pathologization leads, often, it isn't helpful, because it categorizes our behavior as "other," instead of helping us become a functional, healthy version of ourselves. Instead of validating her lived experience, those messages ultimately made her question if she only liked sex because she was assaulted. She became focused on these outside messages instead of getting in touch with how she actually felt about her own sexuality. Looking outward can be useful, and finding helpful sources of sexual education can be helpful, but without being centered in how we feel and what we want, those influences can be distracting, or even damaging.

Media representations and discussions of sex after sexual assault frequently portray survivors as one of two stereotypes: promiscuous, unhealthily risk-driven, sex-obsessed; or celibate, broken, afraid of sex. Other factors can complicate this false binary. In reality, it's not a choice between two extremes, but more like a spectrum. This is true of any sexual stereotype: promiscuous/prudish; Madonna/whore; dom/sub; top/bottom. Most people fall somewhere in the middle, or shift throughout their lives. Plus, broad categories like "risky" evoke stereotypes, not realities. What constitutes a risk for one person may be a requirement for somebody else. Few aspects of sex are by definition "risky," and everybody tolerates and negotiates actual risk individually.

A few times in my life, I found myself single and sleeping around more than many of my friends expected of me. I slept with people I met in bars, on dating apps, in hostels, while traveling, through classmates, at parties. I liked meeting new partners and trying new things with them, sexually and socially—like trying on different hats to see which one fits best. To some people, sleeping around evokes a laundry list of new partners, but to me, sleeping around is at least as much about putting myself in different sexual scenarios to better understand who I am. Partners change, but I'm always present when I'm having sex.

If it weren't for my slutty phases—which one of my friends refers to as "data collection"—I wouldn't know as much about my boundaries, desires, or communication preferences. But at other points in my life, I've been in monogamous relationships or single and celibate. Not only do I fall somewhere in the middle of all these sexual spectrums, I also move along them, changing my position over time.

Like me, Alisa doesn't think the promiscuous/prudish divide serves or represents her lived experience. "I have found great healing in intentionally abstaining from sex," Alisa says, continuing, "and I found great healing from having a bunch of sex with some random-ass people." She explains she isn't just promiscuous or prudish. Like me, she feels she's both, at different times throughout her life. In particular, Alisa points to messaging that survivors "have daddy issues all the time, and that they're easy to have sex with." These messages made her feel trapped in society's expectations, but also lost, because they didn't match her lived experience. She felt pressured to heal within a relationship, but recovering from sexual assault in a partnered context—living in a very active "in progress" state—comes with its own set of challenges.

Alisa explains that what we learn through socialization, as well as through our culture and the messaging we receive through the news, makes us feel alone and wrong. "Survivors are stigmatized and shamed for what we've been through and how we heal and how we survive," Alisa says. It's not just about the trauma, it's about how we cope with it too. "Dating is a nightmare whether you have trauma or not . . . sleeping with strangers, sleeping with people we know, it doesn't matter. Or not having sex at all. All that is complicated, for everyone." She acknowledges that yes, survivors have added layers of complexity. "But once we peel back the shame and self-blame, I think there's a lot of compassion for ourselves available to just be like, 'it's okay to be alive and to be messy and to want whatever we want.'" There is so much outside shame and blame that it can be hard to locate what about our sexuality feels authentic to us.

People of diverse genders may face different stereotypes—including men. Through her work as a consent educator, Stacey observes stigma around men experiencing pain and trauma. Stacey points out that if we're so uncomfortable with male or masculine pain as a whole, men are going to have a hard time getting help after trauma, or talking about it. "Being victimized destroys their masculinity," Stacey observes. She thinks that part of this is because if you live on the feminine side of the gender binary, there's almost built-in sympathy for trauma because people expect it to happen to you. But if you fall outside that box of femininity, you don't get the appropriate support.

Stacey gives the example of men in fraternities—hypermasculine spaces—that define their identity, social community, and even personality. Within those organizations, which are responsible for facilitating sexual violence against nonmembers, sexual abuse is also used to control one another's masculinity. Hazing and organized sexual violence occur, but after years of studying and working on campuses, Stacey has observed that fraternity brothers struggle to claim the title of trauma victim. Often they are forced to reconcile with the idea that this trauma forms part of their core identity.

Stacey feels that in the United States, society has progressed enough for her to adopt traditionally masculine attributes. But the reverse doesn't work; she notices men around her unable to access femininity or feminine attributes without being socially punished. "We haven't created enough space for that," she says. The same applies to men who have experienced sexual violence. Stacey sees them have to suffer in silence much of the time, never receiving support to heal from trauma. This extends into how men heal sexually post-trauma—or don't.

"Men in general aren't given license to feel their feelings," Mason, a bisexual man, says. He wishes more men who've experienced assault could express their emotions, have safe places to go to excise disappointment, frustration, and rage, so they don't end up being radicalized by the internet into committing acts of violence. Mason feels he hasn't been given archetypes to live up to of men who are processing emotions and showing their feelings in a healthy space. He sees male sexuality as intrinsically tied to the ego. Men, in Mason's eyes, "define their masculinity by their sexual prowess, whether it's in the bedroom or being able to get somebody into the bedroom." If male sexuality becomes fractured in some way, like through sexual assault, that can "get really fucked up, really, really fast." Lacking access to sources of support that promote healthy masculinity has made it difficult for Mason, like many other male survivors, to heal.

Much of our behavior post-assault is shaped by aspects of our lives completely unrelated to assault, like gender roles, parental relationships, or early access to information about sex. While popular narratives suggest survivors' whole sexual paradigm is defined by our experience of trauma, we are just as multifaceted as our sexual and personal histories. We are affected by sexual experiences, but also by the way sex and relationships were presented to us as kids, as role modeled by adults and peers. And while learning about the ins and outs of sex itself is important, messages we absorb about what a healthy relationship looks like should be paid close attention to, both in understanding our trauma histories and in forming future healthy relationships.

Mason was raised in a deeply conservative, Christian household. He spent a lot of his education in gifted children programs, and felt like he couldn't relate to kids his own age. He ended up being abused by somebody who took advantage of that feeling of isolation. He didn't feel like he could talk to his parents about the abuse or how it affected him. That early exposure to sex acts, even though they were abusive, made him feel like his sexual education happened backward—he did things before he knew what they were, let alone why they felt bad.

Mason recalls his father driving him back from a hockey tournament. Sitting side by side in his dad's car, they didn't make eye contact. His dad broke the silence, saying only, "Do you know about this sex stuff?" Mason effectively shut down the conversation—and that was it. He didn't talk about sex with his parents again at all. He described this to me as a "pretty standard Midwestern sexual education." By the time they started sex ed as a school subject, Mason had already been watching MTV and HBO late-night shows, informally exposing him to another form of sex ed—one meant for entertainment, not education. "I feel like I was warped from the very beginning," Mason says. He, like many young people, had a lot of exposure to sexuality and sexual content before he was really in charge of his own sexual agency.

Over the course of many conversations with his peers, Mason has observed that he tends to be a lot more sexual than the average friend. Whether that's jerking off fifteen times in a day, sleeping around more, or wanting more sex from a partner—he feels he isn't "normal." He's experienced a disconnect between his lived experience and what other people consider normal, and it's left him feeling othered even amongst loved ones. But Mason has begun to accept his sexuality for what it is, and stop comparing it to what other people consider normal.

While Mason is more in tune with his sexuality and accepting of his desires and boundaries than previously, he receives a lot of pressure from partners to perform sexually in a certain way. "Because I'm this big giant guy," Mason says, "a traditionally masculine guy, like I'm fairly hairy and tall . . . it seems like the women that are attracted to me always want me to dominate them, and to be very aggressive, very toppy." But Mason isn't really into that kind of sex. He wants to "do the tender, soft, loving sort of thing," but for decades, no woman wanted that from him.

At this point Mason feels trained to act the way women want him to, and he does enjoy pleasing partners, but it isn't his preference. Today, when Mason is able to break out of that very specific sexual role, it feels amazing—revolutionary. While Mason doesn't feel comfortable with the overall dynamic of being women's "dumb daddy," a hypermasculine dominant role, it's led him to explore a variation he loves: focusing on giving partners pleasure. That style of sex leaves him fulfilled, and gives him pleasure, too. Survivors I've spoken to consistently describe that process of locating our preferred sexual roles, and acting them out, as liberating. Sometimes it's difficult to explain our desire for a certain role to other people. When trying to explain why being submissive during sex feels good to me, I compare it to a scenario many of us face: trying to pick a restaurant to get take-out from with a group. It can get aggravating, go in circles, and feel like nobody's ever going to eat—and you give up on advocating for whatever it is you really want. The group comes to an impasse. Then, somebody steps in and takes charge. They might say, "This is where we're going, end of discussion." Not only is the debate over, a relief, but that dominant person both figured out and picked the restaurant you wanted all along. Being a sub is exactly like that feeling, amplified times a thousand. A dominant partner isn't just there to make all the decisions, they're there to take the reins and guide you through a sexual experience based on what you both want. Using this metaphor has helped me break through some barriers with partners and friends around explaining my sexual interests.

When I meet a new partner for the first time, without me saying anything about my wants or boundaries, I notice their inclination is to treat me like a "good girl." Sometimes, sexual partners actually call me that. The term usually connotes being someone who follows the rules, is submissive, and has a virginal quality—or, at least, an innocent and limited sexual history. This definition is at odds with my actual sexual history and preferences. Like Mason, I have a complicated role with the sexual persona other people force on me. I am small, sometimes quiet, and do tend to play a submissive role during sex. But I also have a long list of ex-partners, like to break the rules and explore my and my partners' kinks, and I am far from "innocent." My lived experience doesn't line up with that descriptor. Sometimes, I choose to play with the sexual role I'm handed, because it can be fun. But understanding it's an influence coming in from the outside helps me stay aware of what I actually want out of sex—not just what I "should" want according to the vibe other people pick up around me. I can play the good girl, but I prefer to think of myself as just a person, figuring out each sexual encounter one at a time. Making individual choices—independent choices, for ourselves—is healing in its own right.

Others' perceptions of our bodies or identities can shape the sex we have. Sometimes, survivors try to alter our bodies to change how partners perceive us. This can come from a place of fear. One survivor I spoke to, Alicia Raimundo, who is nonbinary and bisexual, wanted their body to look "the opposite" of how it appeared at the time of their assault. So they intentionally gained weight, cut and dyed their hair, and got a tattoo. However, their plan backfired; cultural expectations about how female-appearing bodies should look made them self-conscious about their body when they did have sex.

Another survivor felt an intense sense of alienation from her body—its appearance, its sensations, even its presence. Sex was off the table if she couldn't live inside her body. Some other survivors feel this as body dysmorphia, or simply dissociating from sex.

For years after she was assaulted, Lexi felt disconnected from her body, unable to read its signals or connect with herself enough to be present during sex. Some of this distrust came from her body's freeze reaction during her sexual assault, when she felt a disconnect between her urge to fight back and her body's paralyzed response. "My body didn't protect me," she reflects, continuing, "I don't trust my body." She felt her nervous system response had let her down. She believes, looking back, she could have physically fought off her attacker, but her body didn't have that response available to her in that moment. She panicked and froze. Her response in the moment led to her mistrusting her body for years, as well as her decision-making.

That distrust seeped into her relationship with food. She turned to binge eating, which Lexi interprets as her body's response to not feeling safe around food. Eventually she learned about intuitive eating, which involves trusting your body, listening to what it's asking for, and then giving it that nourishment. So, she kept the foods she craved in the house at all times: doughnut holes, Oreos, cookie dough. She encouraged herself to eat anything that had previously felt unsafe to eat, which helped her recalibrate her relationship with her body. This helped her learn to trust that her body knows what it wants, and she should act on how she feels. Lexi's healing work began mostly when she started repairing her relationship with her own body. Talking about what happened wasn't the same.

Matthew, a gay man, experienced body image issues that originated in his childhood. He grew up "gay in a very conservative household, where we don't talk about feelings so much, where we self-soothed with food." He remembers a lot of shame around body and body image. His parents put him on WeightWatchers when he was thirteen years old. He was not out to his family until he was twenty-three, and Matthew felt like he needed to do everything his family wanted to be accepted by them. His body image got tied up in his sexuality, and his desire for approval of both. This created issues later on, after he was sexually assaulted.

By that time, Matthew internalized the idea that his value came from his appearance. He was assaulted by somebody he considered hot, which left him with a harmful message: He wasn't attractive enough for the assailant to consider him an equal, for the assault to have instead been a real relationship. "For a long time I believed that I was the problem because I wasn't good enough for him in a lot of different ways. That took a very long time to unwind." Immediately after the assault, Matthew saw his assailant as "the paragon of, or the arbiter of, value." Ultimately, this left Matthew feeling worthless. It took weekly therapy for years for Matthew to begin to cope with these misperceptions.

Matthew's assault happened soon into his coming out journey. He feels like many of his early sexual experiences, following the assault, might have been better and his learning curve might have been easier had he not been assaulted. There were a lot of aspects of sex that he was still figuring out, like what he enjoyed and who he wanted to sleep with. The assault interrupted the healthy trajectory of that exploration.

Mia was first sexually assaulted while she was a freshman at a small, mostly white liberal arts college. She had existing self-image issues about not being "thin and white and blond" that layered on top of her childhood struggles, being a Black girl adopted into a white family in a largely white town. Her sexual assault occurred in a context in which she already felt she had less value because she was Black. She actually looked up to her assailant, and it took years for her to see him for what he was: a very average man who committed a crime. But she spent years feeling inferior, the crushing weight of racist stereotypes keeping her from having a clear view of what happened and her own self-worth.

Of course, Mia is not the only survivor I spoke to who has struggled with self-worth after assault. At the beginning of the healing process, many of us may be having a hard time with self-worth as a result of trauma. Lyndsey Murray, a straight woman, grew up in Texas in a community where sex ed was virtually nonexistent. The message she received was to abstain until marriage, and she had no real education about how to locate her own or understand others' boundaries. She recognizes, looking back, that she had wanted to stop some of her teenage hookups earlier than she did. But she learned from experience, and over time got better at both recognizing and asserting those boundaries. She remembers arriving at the conclusion, "I need to say something. I deserve to say something." Later, after a sexual assault, her issues with asserting her boundaries in sexual settings intensified. She began having trouble stating and enforcing boundaries in relationships in general, not just during sex, and her crumbling self-worth made it even more difficult to stand up for herself. Her journey took place while she sought out training and ultimately became a sex therapist.

Lyndsey points out that setting boundaries around sex is more difficult than a normal conversation. Speaking from her experience as a straight woman who has been sexually assaulted, she says, "Men can be scary. If you say no, you risk getting hurt because you said no." Lyndsey is referring to how, if she says nothing, a partner can't cross a line, since it hasn't been articulated. If she says no, a partner can choose to ignore it, making the interaction clear-cut sexual assault. It's a view that's shared with other survivors. The only issue we can control, though, is our choice of partner: If we choose partners we trust to listen to us, we can use communication skills to navigate out of any danger zones. If we don't trust a partner to listen, it's important to recognize that as a red flag and act accordingly.

Sometimes survivors' ability to heal after assault is affected by ongoing health issues and mental illness. Survivors I spoke to attributed everything from STDs to ovarian cysts to meningitis as a result of sexual assault as related to the healing process. But mental illness can play a particularly difficult role. Lexi was undiagnosed at the time she was sexually assaulted—it would be years before she would have answers about her ADHD and autism diagnoses. Those factors play a big role in social norms and missing cues, which contributed to getting overwhelmed and being alone and vulnerable to attack when she was assaulted.

It's not uncommon for survivors to begin questioning their sexual orientation or gender identity following an assault. While some outsiders may believe this means sexual assault changes our sexual orientation, actually—as in my experience, coming out as bi—it is a matter of struggling to express who we really are, even as trauma may be working against us.

Alisa, the childhood sexual trauma educator and author, points out that many people are seeking out "explanations" for the queerness of trans and queer survivors, as though those are not natural states of being and require an explanation. Queerness isn't manufactured from trauma, but might be better integrated into our identity as we explore our sexuality post-trauma, and some survivors may become more aware of aspects of our sexuality that we had previously ignored. Plus, the fact that queer and trans kids are more likely to experience sexual harm may contribute to this stereotype.[1]

Although bisexual, Mia stopped sleeping with men for a while after a sexual assault. She felt she couldn't relax into pleasure with a man—basically, that men weren't trustworthy sexual partners. I spoke to her over a period of five years, and during our last conversation, she explained that recently, she's returned to dating mostly men. This fluctuation between preferred gender of a partner is common among sexual assault survivors, and a strong preference for one over the other shouldn't necessarily be viewed as a definitive, lifelong preference.

Mia has noticed another criteria emerging: She tends not to date people who have their own sexual trauma histories, and has noticed women and nonbinary people she's hooked up with and dated do tend to have those histories. She knows, from having difficult conversations herself, how challenging it can be to be the partner of somebody with sexual trauma, and she is aware she might not be able to take on that work in a relationship on top of the work of being a sexual trauma survivor in that same relationship. I find Mia's perspective refreshingly honest. Everybody is entitled to define their own needs and deal-breakers, including wanting to start a relationship with any chosen dynamic.

Laura, an asexual straight woman who was working as a reporter abroad at the time she was raped, remembers how her own identity changed after the assault. "No longer was I 'girl reporter,'" she says, "I was, 'oh my God, the girl who's been gang-raped.'" That was even the newspaper headline used to describe the crime. "It was like a spaceship landed in my life," Laura reflects about how she had to reorient herself toward survival in the aftermath of the rape. Laura identifies on the asexuality spectrum, something consistent since before she was raped. "I've never particularly liked sex," Laura explains, "and as soon as the emotional connection isn't there, I'm kind of like, oh, I don't want to do this anymore." It can feel like a chore. She sees the discrepancy in desire between her and her current partner, her husband, as a direct result of the rape—a lot has become tied up in how she sees sex with her husband that isn't about her baseline asexuality. She feels constant pressure to be sexual with him that makes it difficult to maintain her boundaries and sense of self, and manage the effects of sexual violence. Many ace survivors I spoke to had trouble delineating where the effect of trauma began and asexuality ended, and struggled to explain their preferences and choices to partners. In general, survivors feel basic aspects of our sexuality, like being ace or being gay, are never "new" post-trauma, but rather previously unexplored, and better understood post-trauma.

Ramona identifies as demisexual, which falls under the asexual umbrella and refers to experiencing attraction after getting to know someone, not based on some initial spark. After experiencing sexual assault, Ramona needs to build a lot of trust with her partner in order to get her libido to "spark." She explains, "If I'm not in a relationship with someone, literally sometimes I forget about sex." Ramona continues, "When I'm not involved with someone, I lose interest in sex pretty quickly. But then, when I am with someone, that desire really skyrockets." That split is common among some demi people, but can be initially confusing to work out, including for Ramona.

These days, Ramona's sexuality waxes and wanes, often in relation to her partner's desire. Today, Ramona is initiating sex with her boyfriend much of the time, and would be happy having more sex than him—a first for her. She feels safe with him—potentially difficult for a sexual assault survivor—and that makes space for her to feel sexual with him. He doesn't push boundaries, and the exploration they do together feels secure. Ramona tells me it feels like "the right time and the right person to explore and be sexual."

For some survivors, identification with different aspects of our sexualities changes over time. Leanna didn't feel strong attraction to anyone until her twenties and wondered if she was asexual. She didn't educate herself on the matter. As she grew up, she noticed herself experiencing more and more attraction to men, realizing "I'm a raging heterosexual!" Overnight, she went from not caring about men around her to, "I can smell hot dudes, this is weird." Leanna learned to accept her new attraction over time. Similarly, Lexi didn't recognize her attraction to women until she was in an open relationship with a partner who chose other people for her to sleep with. Lexi came to understand she was bisexual. She had noticed her attraction to women before but never acted on it or thought much about it. Post-assault, inside this healing but difficult relationship dynamic, Lexi found room to broaden her sexuality.

A lot of survivors I spoke to acknowledged that if they'd had better sex education as children—both relating to sexual assault and sex in general — they would have felt better equipped to navigate their trauma later on in life. Lexi points out that sexual assault is a common experience among teenagers, but without sex ed about it, or even talking to a trusted adult about how to navigate that aspect of becoming intimate with somebody, young people are left to navigate the world by trial and error. The error can be extremely harmful. She in particular wishes sex ed taught that sexual assault was common enough that you might experience it, and also what to do not only during an assault but how to deal with it afterward. It's not enough to teach only about positive outcomes, since many people have their sexuality weaponized against them. Education about our bodies and sexual preferences should start from a young age, regardless of whether or not you've been assaulted.

Even though he grew up in a very progressive state, the hometown Matthew grew up in had an abstinence education–only policy at his public school in the mid 2000s. "We got education on STDs, and that was it," he says. He explains he doesn't remember them talking about consent, but if they did, it did not feel relevant to his sex life because he was still in the closet at that point, and the sex ed was mostly about straight sex.

Matthew learned about sex from other sources. His dad spoke to him vaguely about it, but didn't leave him with any answers, only a lot of shame around sex and sexuality. "Most of what I learned growing up was from the internet," Matthew says. He first found porn online in sixth or seventh grade, which was the first time he felt he was getting substantial information about sex. Porn gave him access to a world of examples he could pick and choose from. Armed with more information, he began to explore his sexuality in the real world.

Some survivors, like Matthew, find porn to be a useful tool to try out sexual scenarios or engage in our own sexuality, without involving another person who might have different desires, expectations, or boundaries. It can be a safe way to engage with our sexuality after assault, whether or not we engaged with it earlier. Being mindful of how porn influences our views on sex and partners can help keep everybody safe.

In fact, Stacey believes that some version of porn-based education could be helpful to all survivors. She wishes survivors of sexual assault could do a flipped version of the SAR she had to do through school: not boundary-pushing content, but "exposure to intimacy and consent, and pleasure and healthy relationships." Whatever you internalized from trauma, whether it was one experience or over an extended period of time, could be denormalized in this kind of group context. "When you come out of it, you feel stronger in your convictions about who you are as a sexual person, relationships and setting boundaries, having conversations," Stacey says. That kind of reassessment of your norms and beliefs can be healing to anybody, offering the idea that sex can be positive. Access to sex ed is inherently empowering, Stacey says.

Growing up in the Unitarian Church, Mia received robust sex ed by the end of eighth grade. "We learned everything, literally everything," Mia recalls, and "there was a whole bit on assault and consent." She reflects that today's rising conversations about consent bring with them the new question of how and when to teach kids about the subject—but Unitarians have been doing it well for a very long time.

Mia went to a parochial boarding school for high school, where she found herself "completely drenched in purity culture." She feels her time at the boarding school undid some of the sex-positive messaging she received through Unitarian sex ed. Juxtaposed with her upbringing in a very liberal family with Catholic origins, Mia struggles to reconcile her different sources of sex education and beliefs. "I didn't grow up in purity culture," Mia explains, "but I adopted it as a teenager, and it lasted into adulthood." It affected how she views sexual assault, explaining that she feels it was her fault because she did something sexual—not only the sexual nature of the relationship she had with her abuser, but also just the fact that she chose to go to his house that night. She questions whether her reaction to the sexual assault and her sexuality in the aftermath would have been different if she hadn't had purity culture beliefs and Catholic reactionary guilt in her. She had been steeped in toxic beliefs around sexuality, and it was only after the assault, and after doing more internal work and exploration with partners, that she began to untangle it all—both the impact of trauma and the influence of purity culture.

Leanna grew up homeschooled in a conservative Christian family. Her mom, a nurse, gave her a clinical lecture on sex and books about puberty, but her exposure to education about her sexuality was limited. Overall, she had very little education around the consequences—emotional or physical—of sex, or pregnancy, or how birth control can affect you. She had no real grounding in the idea that a romantic relationship could lead to sex, and that having sex without protection could lead to pregnancy. Leanna didn't seek out more information on her own—it was the unknown unknown—and she didn't become sexually active until her early twenties.

Not long after, she was sexually assaulted. The assault doubled her existing difficulties with sex, and she avoided sexual experiences moving forward for a long time. She'd had a sexual partner before the assault—not a very satisfying relationship, she explains, but she was being active. Like Matthew, she feels the trauma delayed what her sexual trajectory might have looked like had she not been assaulted.

After the assault, Leanna suffered from a lot of PTSD symptoms. She tried to avoid sex, and when she did engage in something sexual with her new partner, she ended up experiencing a lot of dissociation and other symptoms. She couldn't engage in sex positively. "I was worried I had multiple personalities," she says, unclear what was happening to her and why she could be so into her new partner but then have to stop sex so often. Leanna, who identifies as a curious person in general, had always been a researcher, so she dove deep into research about how it was impacting her sexuality. Her sexual education, so lacking in childhood, became a new, post-trauma project. She experimented with what she liked and didn't like, and how triggers affected her sex life. But she always kept in mind her baseline, checking in with herself about whether what she was doing felt good or not.

Many people coming out of recent trauma can't even imagine what their life will be like ten years in the future. Leanna, who is now ten years out from experiencing trauma, sees that she spent the first five years "very much in survival mode." PTSD symptoms she didn't expect kept popping up and she had to address them as they came. Some survivors in Leanna's position avoid dating altogether because it can help you avoid negative feelings when you're just starting to feel better post-assault. Dating may not be the priority, depending on where a survivor is at. This part of healing might come later—like for Leanna, who feels that it is only more recently, in the past five years, she has been developing better techniques, fine-tuning her self-care, and focusing on sex in a way that feels like more than just keeping her head above water.

After a childhood steeped in conservative Christian values, Ramona took it upon herself to do her own research about sex. Struggling with sexual trauma as well as gynecological health conditions, she reads articles, watches YouTube videos from sex therapists or people into BDSM or kink. Many sexual assault survivors, like Ramona and Leanna, go through a reeducation related to sex. Often, not only was their sex education growing up inadequate, it also made their post-traumatic experiences more difficult or even painful.

Ramona's early sex ed came partly from sex scenes in movies, but she became critical of what she was seeing later on in life. She thinks, off the top of her head, about a "dumb movie," a rom-com, about a sexually charged relationship between two people who supposedly hate each other. In the scene, the characters used a condom, and Ramona likes how this is becoming normalized. But she points out they didn't use any lube. "We're still shown a lot of things in social media and media that are not indicative of how sex actually goes," Ramona says.

"It's totally normal to have to stop and use lube, or to maybe use a toy, or to need more foreplay before sex, or whatever it is." Ramona recognizes the differences between sex on screen and sex in real life, and the positive impact of normalizing real life safer sex.

Many survivors are taking stock of our sexual needs and wants as impacted by our trauma histories, beyond those initial learnings from sex ed and early life. Where we are right now, today, affects what we want—and we don't need to pressure ourselves to want a different sexual identity or sex life than what we need in this moment. These things evolve, but only we are qualified to be honest about our own feelings, comfort level, and desire. In the stories of our sexual lives, we are character, narrator, and writer, defining the plot and who we want to become. The decisions are up to us.

But we don't exist in a vacuum, and we can call on others to support us. Moving forward, it's important to take stock of what sources of support we have access to as we work to become the most authentic versions of our sexual selves.

CHAPTER 3

We Heal in Community

I HAVE DEALT with sexual assault while thousands of miles from home, shortly after a move and with little social support. Where in the past, during a crisis, I may have reached out to my mom or my best friend to help "coordinate" my care, or at least check in on me regularly—reminding me to reach out to a therapist and eat regularly—I found myself totally isolated. I realized I would have to lean on myself as the center of my support system. I would have to coordinate the crisis—but I wouldn't have to do it in isolation. I asked a friend to come over the day after I was assaulted, and she took me grocery shopping. Another friend let me talk it out and take a nap on his couch. And I found a support group to participate in when I felt totally adrift. It was tough—much tougher than when I had been assaulted in the past and had local friends and family to support me. But ultimately, even when I've healed from assault with support, I know I can't get better without captaining the ship myself, because only I know what I really need.

It takes more than one supportive friend, one therapist, or one understanding partner to heal from sexual assault and build a healthy sex life. It takes us, as survivors, advocating for ourselves at every step of the way. Many survivors I spoke to immediately mentioned their partner when talking about the support they could access when dealing with fallout from sexual violence. But not everybody has a partner at the time they are assaulted, and many survivors with partners find those partners' reactions to be less than supportive. Some people have success with supportive therapists, but others find therapists don't work out well. Understanding the context of social support in which we are each healing is an important step toward figuring out what we want sexually, post-assault.

The context in which we heal is shaped partly by language. The words we have available to describe our experiences of trauma determine how we talk about what happened to us—and the terms we have in our arsenal to describe our sex lives and relationships affect how we approach the two. Terms like "ghosting" or "breadcrumbing" mean something different from breaking up or being inconsistent, and "love bombing" or "gaslighting" aren't quite the same as manipulation. Being surrounded by therapy-speak isn't necessarily helpful when we seek out therapy. Nobody heals in a vacuum even when we're alone, because we think about healing using language other people came up with, popularized, and used. As we seek to describe our needs and issues to other people, it's helpful to stay aware of the language we use, and reach for terminology that will help.

Lexi tells me that just how trauma tends to involve somebody else, healing happens in community too. Lexi calls this community-dependent healing "co-regulation," something she learned in somatics coaching school. We can help each other regulate—especially our partners. So how do you set up relationships for success, or help your partner hold you, ground you? Many people expect survivors to show up to relationships or dating fully healed. We're not supposed to engage at all until we're "ready." This mindset is black and white, and not that helpful.

Lyndsey observed that questions around the impact of trauma on sex are complex, not only through personal experiences but also through her work as a sex therapist. We don't show up at any particular moment as our full sexual selves—our experiences shape us throughout our life. Family dynamics in childhood, our cultural background, messages we receive around sex growing up, vulnerabilities that affect our healing processes—all of these can impact our sexuality and sexual healing processes by the time we are sexually assaulted or begin to heal. Lyndsey says that being queer, kinky, or polyamorous can affect who we are and how we heal too. The idea that there is no "true" self to return to complicates healing, explaining that she struggled with the idea that "there's something wrong with me if I don't go back to how things were." There is no return, only deepening our understanding of where we are now, and how that context might enable us to grow from here. These questions extend into her work as a sex therapist, too.

Mia clearly describes to me how her healing process has been affected by factors outside the sexual assault itself—especially being a Black woman who was adopted transracially. Mia says that people have this "image of the sexual assault victim being this battered woman." She finds this harmful because it takes away victims' agency beyond the experience of the assault itself. If she goes into a sexual encounter disclosing she has been assaulted but doesn't act very affected by it, other people act like they think something is wrong with her, "because you need to be broken, or else it's not real." Mia underscores that "our stereotype of women in particular after sexual assault is really detrimental because it doesn't allow victims to be strong people who are okay." There isn't room for healing at the pace Mia feels most comfortable with. She notes that "at the same time, specifically in the Black community, Black women are expected to get up and keep going." Within that community specifically, allowing people to be wounded is important, but "woundedness shouldn't be a requirement" for people after they've been assaulted. Mia wants more space to define for herself what post-traumatic growth can look like, beyond the expectations of her community.

At the time she was raped, Mia was primarily immersed in white culture. Since she was adopted, growing up, and into her early adulthood, she didn't have strong Black role models to look up to, especially when it came to healthy relationships. Until she was in college, she only saw Black adults in Black nativity, or moms whose kids' dads were absent. She never saw herself represented in a healthy relationship until she was grown up. Her role models of women dating women were similarly skewed: While lesbian role models allowed her to see representation outside of straight culture, she noticed particular examples of Black lesbian women she knew moving quickly into relationships and then crashing and burning, or Black women in very serious relationships for years without healthy boundaries or intentionality. Mia feels that the lack of healthy role models influenced her to keep sleeping with her rapist on and off for months after the assault. She felt she had no positive example to aspire to. Being in communities that give us access to role models, and helping form a supportive context in which to heal, can completely change a survivor's outlook on their own life.

About a year after the rape, Mia got in touch with her birth mother, looking for support. But her birth mother didn't want to have contact with her at that time, because, as she told Mia "a step above implied and a step below explicitly stated," Mia was a product of rape. It was the most devastating part of their interaction, and for all the progress Mia had made since her sexual assault, she felt that this new pain related to her birth mother "replaced the pain of someone taking my agency away." She felt inundated by sexual violence, and finding her birth mother, something she had hoped would be healing, caused fresh pain. Mia had thought she was headed in the direction of healing, but life is not neat, and it's impossible to tell exactly what our healing efforts will yield. Unfortunately, Mia's step forward ended up feeling like several steps back. Mia experienced compounding difficulty while trying to recover from sexual trauma, an experience shared by many, if not most, survivors.

Leanna, who experienced PTSD symptoms for two years without reaching out for trauma-specific help, became pregnant early into her first real relationship after she was assaulted. She decided to continue the pregnancy and put her child up for adoption. It wasn't until after this second crisis that Leanna felt she was in an emotionally safe place to go through therapy for her sexual assault. Her therapist, whom she was referred to through her adoption agency, specialized in CBT and worked with her not only on PTSD but also post-adoption grief and depression. They focused a lot on short-term survival skills: coping with suicidality, maintaining a healthy baseline. Leanna applied those concepts to her longer-term recovery, too.

Leanna's sexual assault trauma layered on top of the difficult emotional and physical experience of carrying a pregnancy and giving a child up for adoption. The compounding traumas speak to a broader theme: We don't heal from sexual assault while, somehow, the rest of our lives are frozen. We are dealing with relationships, family emergencies, work stress, moving across the country, caregiving duties, medical issues—the list is endless, because sexual assault doesn't preclude us from experiencing further life difficulties. And for many of us, even without additional stressors, our "normal" routine may become a minefield of triggers—interacting with people who are the same gender as our attacker, having to be in crowded spaces or deal with loud noises, or simply being unable to function as normal because of traumatic stress. We don't get to go on a healing retreat and come out cured. But we can make use of the resources available to us—sometimes, including resources relating to compounding issues, like Leanna's adoption process.

Leanna also learned a lot from the birth parent community. They taught her to listen to her gut. She noticed that if her anxiety rises a lot, she gets strong, pulsing stomachaches. Today, she asks her gut questions, and when it clenches, she can intuit where her anxiety might be coming from. Leanna has made a point of learning how trauma physically manifests in her own body, using the resources made available to her after life got even more complicated. The connection between physical symptoms and PTSD is well-documented, and Leanna's ability to get in touch with her body's response to triggers and challenges helps her navigate life.[1] These skills directly translate into how she approaches checking in with her body during sex today. Healing happens while the rest of your life is happening.

Right before Lyndsey took her final exams and got certified to be a therapist, a friend sexually assaulted her. At the time of the assault, Lyndsey was in a relationship, and her immediate sexual response was "totally freaking out when having sex." She left the partner she was with at the time of the assault, then quickly started dating somebody new. Lyndsey did what many sexual assault survivors are encouraged to do: seek refuge from trauma in a relationship, with a partner.

It didn't work. Her new partner was unsupportive of her healing process, and made her feel guilty for setting sexual boundaries. Sex became mired in anxiety, even though she knew, both as an individual and a freshly minted sex therapist, that sex was something you were supposed to enjoy. She had to do a lot of work around it: what was happening in her body and mind, how to address it, and how to communicate with her partner about it. "It's kind of like reorienting yourself," Lyndsey says. Lyndsey broke up with her post-assault partner after he pushed too many of her boundaries, and ultimately found that healing alongside a partner is only beneficial if that partner is supportive. A lot of healing work can happen alone or in nonsexual relationships—and it can't happen in a relationship that is harmful.

Some sexual assault survivors I spoke to took a broad view of healing in the context of the real world—a world that can prove dangerous. We may be healing from particular assaults, but we also live in a world that puts us at high risk of further violence. Ramona describes her survivor identity as "someone who is experiencing sexual assault" because she sees her life that way: even when she is not being assaulted, she consistently has her physical and sexual boundaries pushed. Ramona has experienced many "low level" sexual assaults, her words for violence that wasn't as far on the spectrum as rape, but her boundaries have been pushed into sexual assault territory. She also recognizes several instances of boundary-pushing in her life that did not result in actual boundary violations, but served to highlight how often boundaries are at risk of being violated. Ramona describes these to me as "moments of discomfort." A consistent theme through her traumatic experiences has been her asserting boundaries and them being ignored—so expected, at this point, that she sees this as inevitable. This runs counter to the idea that if we ask for what we want, we can prevent our own assaults. She views those violations as an expected part of existing in the world and navigating relationships.

Ramona feels empathy for women who don't want men in their lives at all, because they just want to cut off the sources of so much pain. She feels she is at a place where she is fighting hard to be in relationships with men, to communicate and push through uncomfortable moments. She sees this work as one-sided much of the time. Ramona wishes that partners of trauma survivors and men, in particular, would be more proactive in supporting victims and helping them feel comfortable, whether that's in a romantic or social relationship. Her current partner has done what she wishes more men would do: take on that responsibility of educating himself about dating and communicating with people with trauma. He took a multipart online course on the subject. She believes traumatized people should not be burdened with educating our partners, ourselves. Rather, they should do the work of learning and unlearning.

Ramona has noticed that when she calls a partner out on pushing a boundary, they'll typically apologize. But she's never gotten an apology from a man who noticed his own bad behavior by himself. She doesn't pay much attention to their apologies at this point simply because it's happened so often. Ramona has rejected many potential partners for threatening behaviors, wary that those smaller threats could escalate into violence or ignored boundaries later on. "It's very hard for me to trust men," Ramona explains, "because I have dated men." Her lived experience dating men, has shaped her attitude about sex and dating, not just the trauma she has experienced. She recognizes that we live in a world where sexual assault can and does happen. Trauma lingers in our bodies, but we can use it as a foundation to build better sexual practices. At this point, relentlessly asserting her boundaries is Ramona's focus. Part of her healing was realizing that what other people do after she expresses a boundary is out of her control. She can't count on any particular partner to be a positive step toward healing, and looks at the bigger picture. Only she can choose her path forward. She can lean on herself for support as she does the work of seeking out support from other people.

Several survivors I spoke to who were in relationships at the time of their assault felt pressured to return to having sex sooner than they were ready. But we never actually owe anybody sex. Laura got into a relationship soon after being assaulted, and ended up in couple's therapy for related issues. Lyndsey broke up with her partner. There are many ways to navigate sex after sexual assault with a partner—many avenues toward stability, safety, and pleasure.

It seems like everybody—friends, doctors, Instagram ads—wants us to get therapy, regardless of if we need it. While therapy can be a useful tool for healing after sexual assault, including as it impacts our sex lives, therapy isn't a great fit for everyone. Ultimately, therapists are human. They can misinterpret what survivors tell them, or ask damaging questions; one therapist suggested I ask myself why I got myself into situations where I ended up a victim of violence (the definition of victim blaming). Lexi says that it's common for high-masking, women-presenting autistic/ADHD people like herself to overintellectualize. When she tried out talk therapy, she ended up running her own therapy session. She felt like she was playing both her role and the therapist's. The therapist didn't have much to offer besides validation, and Lexi felt like she wasn't getting anything out of her sessions. Support systems popular today, like talk therapy, aren't a good fit for everybody. So, Lexi turned to nontraditional methods to heal her relationship with her body, including intuitive eating. She joined women's circles that practiced deep pelvic breathing and yoni massages, teaching her to reconnect to her body with other women as witnesses and supportive guides.

While many survivors feel that we are our own best advocates in the healing process, Lexi is wary of our culture's constant critiquing of codependency. She believes it makes more sense to think of ourselves as dependent on other people. We're social creatures. Our physical well-being depends on our social context and our access to social support. "Having needs doesn't make you needy," Lexi says. Just because one particular person can't or won't meet your needs doesn't mean it's wrong to have them. Lexi sees a long line of people, especially women, supporting one another across history, right up to the present day. "So to expect," Lexi says, "that we go and heal [trauma] on our own, or just heal with one therapist, that you're paying for—that is such a harmful narrative." Lexi thinks therapists or coaches can be positive influences, but she has observed that the actual healing happens in her day-to-day life: in practice. Her healing happened with her partners, with women friends, exploring sexually alone, and in community, with partners and peers.

It's not just partners or therapists that can help us heal. I always joke that "friends help friends have good sex," but when it comes to healing from sexual trauma, I think it's actually true. Having people to talk openly with about difficulties in our sex lives opens up our thinking, too. Months after a sexual assault, I chose to tell my close girlfriends I had a crush on a man I was getting to know—whom I knew was interested in me. Even though these friends all knew about the recent assault, they didn't seem to understand where I was coming from when it came to the new guy. Instead of encouraging me to continue connecting with somebody romantically and sexually, they told me to stop seeing him because they didn't think he would make a good life partner for me. They even made fun of his weaknesses (broke, flaky) in an effort to get me to jump ship. Their criticism of my choice of partner made me feel terrible and isolated, and I stopped talking to those friends about anybody else I was interested in.

My goal, though, had nothing to do with finding a life partner. I was just proud of myself for being vulnerable with somebody. Sometimes, after we are assaulted, we're just trying to get back out there, and finding somebody who feels safe and shows interest are the two main checkboxes. Whether or not somebody we sleep with after assault is our future life partner is often not a concern. Since it's easy to misunderstand what our goals are, it's helpful if both friends of survivors and survivors try to communicate clearly about not just who we're interested in or what we're interested in doing, but why. Surviving sexual assault can change what you're looking for in a partner—or whether you're looking for a partner at all. Friends can build a better understanding that survivors' needs might be different than what they used to be.

I'm not the only one who's shied away from talking about an assault or my later sexual choices to friends. Stacey didn't tell many friends about her abusive ex. She texted a single friend when she was in danger while leaving her ex, and that friend reached out to a few others out of concern. One friend let her stay in her house to get away from her partner, where her ex was less likely to go looking for her. But overall, her friends respected her privacy and let her decide how much to tell them. Her friends have been with her for over a decade, and they have an unspoken agreement that if something bad happens in any of their lives, they can talk about it or not. But no matter how much or little she chooses to share, Stacey knows she will receive support. The overall attitude that sharing was welcome but *not* sharing wasn't a reason for her friends to be unsupportive, is something Stacey has tried to learn from and act on when people approach her with stories about their own trauma history.

Leanna had a friend group in adolescence that mostly consisted of people who happened to have been sexually assaulted. She watched how trauma affected them, how they coped with it, how it colored their personalities, and the way it changed how they thought about their future. Leanna's own sexual assault was attempted but not completed, and she wasn't raped. The trauma stayed with her and is present in her body. But having grown up around sexual assault survivor friends, she felt it was hard to accept her own assault, since it hadn't technically ended in rape. For a long time she said she had been mugged, not sexually assaulted, focusing on the charges she knew she could defend—in Leanna's case, robbery and battery. "It didn't look like what my friends experienced," Leanna says, expressing confusion over whether she should be grateful she hadn't been raped, sorry for her own experience, or rejected by her community because it wasn't "bad enough" (even though none of her friends took that angle). While Leanna's friends may seem like an obvious source of support, her confusion over the details of the assault made her hesitant to rely on them. Every survivor's experience is different, though, and it can be helpful to people in Leanna's position to focus on what the impact of the assault was. We aren't all assaulted in the same way, but much of the time the experience of trauma overlaps, like symptoms of PTSD that Leanna shared with her friends.

Mason survived sexual assault as a kid. For a long time he didn't consider what happened to him to be sexual assault. Later on, in talking to a therapist and friends in college and beyond, he realized the power dynamic was so off that what happened to him counted as sexual abuse. Having people around to validate his experience untangling his memories proved instrumental in recognizing his trauma for what it was. He had "hypercompartmentalized" his childhood abuse and hadn't made connections between how it affected his sexuality and sex life for a very long time. It was only in conversation with friends and a therapist that he was able to start to untangle it.

Mason didn't realize the ways in which he was different until he started having candid conversations about sex with people he knew. He realized he viewed sex differently. Only when he was around the LGBTQ+ community did Mason feel some of the tension in his shoulders unwind. He felt that gay peers "got it" in a way other people didn't, because he didn't have to explain his bisexuality to them, a layer that some people got stuck on when Mason tried to talk about assault. He could heal in community with other queer people.

Other than those early experiences disclosing his trauma history, Mason has felt overwhelmingly isolated—with a couple of exceptions. Mason's best friend can empathize with his experience as a closeted bisexual man, even if that friend didn't have the same trauma backstory. Building bridges around commonalities can be helpful if a friend hasn't experienced sexual assault themself, but you have something related to dating or sex in common. An empathetic ear can make a world of difference after experiencing trauma, which is inherently isolating and cuts us off from our communities.

On the other hand, Mason has felt rejected time and again by communities of sexual assault survivors, which should have welcomed him and helped him heal. In fact, he identifies more closely with the experience of isolation than the experience of feeling held by community. A couple of times he has found himself in groups of people, most often women, talking about sexual assault. When he's tried to "chime in," the attitude from the groups has been to silence him, making him feel like these survivors didn't care about what happened to him. "If someone's not willing to give you the floor, give you the space, or to ask a sensitive question, or basically show that secondary level of interest, then it doesn't feel like you're really being listened to," Mason says. Any responses that were superficially supportive that he has gotten through the sexual assault survivor community have felt perfunctory at best. They never invited him to share more. Mason leaves those groups and situations when that happens, to protect himself. By keeping him from sharing his sexual assault history instead of validating it, those people's words only furthered the shame and aloneness Mason has had to deal with throughout his life.

Mason finds, when he can't access social support, that he can take charge of his own well-being. In these situations, he practices mindfulness, because it allows him to not identify too much with his ego or brain or even his experiences, and observe his thoughts in a more detached way. That is how he stays present, and he thinks it's more helpful than getting strongly identified with trauma, or paying attention to what other people have to say about it. He sees people he knows get stuck in trauma and find it difficult to shake it off and grow. He sees trauma as living in the past, and moving past it is about living in the present. It was helpful for him to let go of those experiences, since he hasn't experienced the option of being supported while experiencing trauma.

While he has limited support from friends and the survivor community, Mason has found a safe haven in his current partner. She reaches out proactively to ask if she's providing the space he needs, and assures him that she loves him—all of him. She asks him follow-up questions and gives him the floor. It's the first time someone other than his best friend has made Mason feel loved and held in that way. Because of his experiences, Mason thinks it's important to find somebody who is willing to hear you out and give you space to talk, whether that's a traditional sexual assault–oriented group or just one of your good friends, or even just yourself, if you're able to hold space for yourself, too. Mason has also discovered that the right people actually want to help, and hiding difficult things from people who love you denies them that opportunity. Good people want to be there for you, even if you find it hard to ask.

Mason has sought out sources of support outside of interpersonal settings. Music helped him feel less alone. The Frank Ocean album *Blonde*, which relates a lot of bi experiences, was the first time Mason had really seen popular media—that all of his friends also knew and loved—directed toward the experience of being bi, like him. It's one of the things that made him realize that representation matters. That proved to be as helpful a resource as any more directly helpful one, because it normalized something difficult in his life. In fact, for a long time Mason didn't know there were other people who had gone through something like him. He didn't know official resources existed. "It's all about finding the right people and finding your community, your place, and your people that will listen and care," Mason says.

In the wake of violence, many survivors turn to medical professionals for support—a step that makes sense, and often does yield assistance. But doctors don't necessarily receive effective training in how to handle sexual assault survivors' treatment, and may even end up doing or saying something harmful.

In health-care settings, Stacey has watched a doctor check a box saying she is a survivor of sexual assault, but then be completely at a loss for how to meet her needs. "They are not trained to have a conversation with you," Stacey says. She wishes doctors would do more education in this area.

When Ramona first saw a physician about her sexual struggles post-assault, she was also just beginning to be sexually active and struggling with vaginismus, a condition that can make sex painful. She had already done research on the issue, and made many attempts to resolve it on her own. She was in the middle of describing to a doctor how she'd already attempted to resolve the issue, and asked this new medical professional if she had any additional advice. "Well, there's this great sex shop," the medical professional began. Ramona was shocked that this was all she offered. She told the doctor, "I know about sex shops—I'm sexually educated." Ramona had come to a professional because Google had failed her, not because she wanted a professional to read out 101 advice to her. "It's very easy for professionals to talk down to you and assume that you don't even know the basics," Ramona says, with the caveat that maybe there are some folks who might need a doctor to give them just the basics. In particular, Ramona is frustrated that she went to a doctor with a medical problem, and the doctor refused to address it from a medical perspective, putting the issue back on Ramona personally. This reflects many sexual assault survivors' experiences, who are left with physical manifestations of trauma, and fail to obtain support through the health-care system. Then, we're pushed away and told the issue will resolve on its own, or that the issue is mostly in our heads—or that the issue isn't an issue at all.

Ramona finds this is especially true of doctors she's seen for her vaginismus, partly because pain can be difficult to communicate about. One day, a new doctor didn't give her off-the-cuff advice without really listening. She sat with Ramona in all her feelings of frustration and disappointment and didn't dismiss her concerns or her sexuality as invalid. A positive experience with a doctor can be life-changing, and Ramona is proof that sexual assault survivors who aren't receiving enough support from their doctor can always look for a new one. Unlike in personal relationships, there might not be room to move forward with a medical professional if they are not well suited to help you.

Ramona has found support in therapists for a long time, since she was five or six years old, she says. She developed the ability to articulate her experiences in a therapy setting early. That proved helpful growing up in a household where "feelings were not okay—the one feeling that was acceptable was anger." Her brother would run away, her mother came from a family that yelled a lot, and Ramona struggled to unpack what was going on while dealing with sexual violations from an early age.

Though she had the support of a therapist, Ramona had more difficulty getting support within her family. When she first tried to disclose a part of her trauma history to her mother, Ramona wasn't able to explain if it was a sexual assault or an uncomfortable sexual situation. Part of Ramona's uncertainty stemmed from the fact that her family members had histories of sexual assault that she felt were more severe than what she had dealt with at that point in her life. Her mother "did not have the language to even talk about her own sexual assault experiences," making the conversation Ramona wanted to have about her own life all but impossible.

Ramona's mom ended up in therapy to wrestle with her early adulthood sexual assaults and a grooming experience similar to what Ramona experienced as a kid. Once her mother better understood her own trauma history, she was able to have more healthy conversations with Ramona, including acknowledging that Ramona's grooming experience "was not safe for you," and apologizing for not protecting her. In order to unlearn some of the negative messages she got from her mother as a child, she had to help her mom unlearn some of those same things, too. Sometimes, in order to cultivate our own supportive communities, we end up having to educate the people we want to hold space for us.

Therapy for post-assault sexual recovery comes with its own set of challenges. In her discussion of a survivor's credibility, trauma expert Judith Herman writes: "When the victim is already devalued (a woman, a child), she may find that the most traumatic events of her life take place outside the realm of socially validated reality."[2] When a sexual assault survivor identifies as a woman, a minor, a person of color, queer, or in another way marginalized, many people fail to listen to us as individuals.

Gabby faced the additional challenges of being a woman of color, Latinx, in a medical environment. Through her university, she found a therapist who understood her experience and her need to reconnect with her body. (Later, Gabby realized how lucky she was to have access to the support of a university counseling system. A few years later, as a young entrepreneur, she bemoaned the lack of support for sexual assault survivors after they leave the university system.) Gabby worked with a therapist who specialized in EMDR, eye movement desensitization and reprocessing therapy. EMDR is a popular treatment for trauma that helps patients process disturbing memories in sync with rhythmic tapping or visuals to draw the eyes to the left and right.[3] This treatment method helped Gabby process her traumatic memories, and its positive impact extended beyond her mental roadblocks to her physical and sexual triggers, too. EMDR changed how Gabby moved through her day-to-day life and how she felt in her body. Though it wasn't the sole focus of her therapy sessions, EMDR improved her sex life.

Therapy also helped Gabby cultivate more sex-positive views. Sex-positivity is an outlook on sex that is supportive, open-minded, and shame-free. It rejects negative views on sex, like that it is dangerous, shameful, or harmful. It was important to Gabby that her partners embrace and live by the same values.

Stacey got in a serious car accident in the process of trying to leave her abusive ex. The doctor who helped her through cognitive rehabilitation after her traumatic brain injury also gave her space for therapy. Stacey says, "I think having someone focus so much on me and my well-being—a stranger" helped flip a switch in her brain that allowed her to come back to herself and what she needed and wanted. She believes without that doctor she wouldn't have had the necessary help to get out of her abusive relationship.

While Stacey, who studied sexuality in graduate school, has found her own education to be immensely therapeutic, she has also engaged in therapy specifically for trauma, including a method called brainspotting. She says that for people with a trauma history or PTSD diagnosis, brainspotting can help process emotions and traumatic experiences in a way that talk therapy or CBT might not. Stacey's therapist held an object, like a pen, and asked her questions continuously while Stacey kept her eyes on the same object. She describes it as a "bizarre out-of-body experience," because while she was processing the emotions, she wasn't able to control them. Typically, her encounters with her emotions left her rigid and unaffected—she wasn't deeply feeling them. But through brainspotting, everything came pouring out. After the sessions, she felt overwhelmed and refused to speak to anybody for the rest of the day, but after a while she felt better—much better. After a few months of this kind of therapy, her whole outlook changed. She still carries the trauma she experienced, and knows it won't ever disappear, but brainspotting helped her access more peace within herself.

Matthew was struggling with the aftermath of assault while simultaneously dealing with an abusive work environment. Juggling both at the same time proved difficult. It felt like there were issues with his life everywhere he turned, and each problem competed for time in therapy. He had worked with the same therapist before the assault and after, over a total of eight years. She noticed something was wrong immediately post-assault, even while he resisted the reality of what he was dealing with. In that immediate aftermath, his therapist recognized that he wasn't ready to face what happened head-on, and they confronted and overcame his trauma together slowly, over time, with a more contained approach. Over the year and a half immediately following the assault, therapy wasn't directly helpful with his trauma, and he focused on other issues with his therapist. But later on, therapy was a useful outlet for him, and while some survivors find therapy frustrating, Matthew felt it was ultimately very helpful.

While I've found that therapists are helpful to my healing, it's mostly supportive community and open lines of communication with loved ones that's proven helpful long-term to me. Building the muscle of talking about the impact of sexual assault is something I can flex if and when there is more trauma fallout, whether because of a circumstantial trigger or later assault. Time and again, though, I find that talking, specifically to other sexual assault survivors, about sex is one of the most powerful means of healing.

The friends I told after I was raped at age eighteen were mostly other teenagers like me. At that age, few of them had experienced sexual assault personally, and not as many people had real empathy compared to when I talk about sexual assault with my current peers, in their thirties. So, I took what friends who *had* experienced sexual assault said seriously. Sometimes, like with my friend Elsa, I took what they said too seriously, and allowed their perspective to stand in for mine. Elsa, a straight woman, had experienced sexual assault as a preteen and later in her early twenties. She believed that when hooking up with somebody, she could say no at any time, and the other person would stop—a faith in humanity (and particularly men) that I would never fully adopt as my own. She trusted near strangers with her body, even if she didn't actually trust them. She felt angry and invincible around men and was experimenting with her desirability as social currency. While none of these behaviors were exclusive to being a trauma survivor, all of them were made more extreme by her trauma history. The world is not as black and white as Elsa painted it for me back then, and it took recovering on my own and with additional sources of support for me to pave my own way forward.

After I made friends with Elsa, I started meeting more sexual assault survivors and, as time went by, became more open about my trauma history with them. We talked about sex and dating just like any friends might, but because of our shared history, it felt like they really *got it*. Eventually, I sought out sexual assault survivor groups and went to events where I was more likely to meet other survivors, like marches and workshops. For me, connecting with other survivors is the most supportive environment in which to heal. Even today, I'm a regular drop-in at my local sexual assault survivor group.

Part of this journey meant figuring out not just what felt safe, but what I wanted—a conversation I've had with many sexual assault survivors, including the ones in the next chapter.

CHAPTER 4

What You Want

HAVING SEX AFTER sexual assault can be exhausting. It feels like project management: a lot of shifting components, as much planning as possible, and then the actual product looks completely different from what you imagined. Sometimes, with the right partner, I find a way around all that juggling: I hand over the reins. Armed with the knowledge of my triggers and boundaries, as well as my desires and sexual interests, I let the right person run the encounter. They choose what we do, for how long, and—unless I say to stop—what to try. This kind of domination allows me to relax into the experience in a way I don't do during vanilla sex, during which I feel the need to constantly check in with myself and the other person, or proactively guide the experience away from triggers. My fantasy will always be to let go of control, into the right person's hands. This doesn't make sense to some people, since sexual assault also involves losing control. But violence happens when somebody else rips away your agency—not when you place it in somebody else's hands yourself. From the outside, these experiences may appear the same, but the internal experience is completely different. If I surrender control to somebody else, it's helpful for me to do a sort of post-game analysis with my partner, a form of intellectual aftercare that soothes my nerves.

Many times, when survivors spoke about how they negotiated power and control with partners, my own experience differed. In particular, I heard many people touch on their experience with consensual nonconsent (CNC) sex, or rape fantasies that they played out in real life. To me, repeating elements of a rape on purpose doesn't feel freeing or empowering. It feels triggering. But since my goal for this book is to normalize the breadth of survivor experiences, I enthusiastically listened to stories far outside the margins of mine.

In a way, fantasies are the opposite of flashbacks. Having a flashback means reliving a traumatic experience as if it were happening again in real time, losing control over your hold on reality and getting caught in the past. Fantasies occur when the brain is a refuge, while flashbacks take place in a brain that morphs into a site of re-traumatization. Fantasies are present- and future-oriented, and allow complete control over your imagination, including envisioned sexual scenarios. When I spoke to survivors, many were interested in how fantasies can be used to explore healing scenarios and use them with a partner or even alone.

If I like someone, I might masturbate while playing out the scene of what it might be like to sleep with them before we ever touch. Exploring a potential sexual relationship in this way feels safer. It functions as exposure therapy, desensitizing me to potential pitfalls and preparing me for what it might feel like. Fantasies aren't reality, though, and I have to remind myself that the other person might have completely different desires and boundaries than I do. I can't fully know what it's like to have sex with someone before actually sleeping with them.

For survivors, fantasies can feel like the inverse of negative reactions to trauma we are burdened with, like flashbacks or nightmares. Starting after she was assaulted as a teenager, Lexi had the same recurring nightmare. She dreamed of a specific subway station in New York City near where she grew up and was assaulted, where she had spent time with her attacker before the assault. The stairs in the subway station felt endless, like she was in the center of the earth. The nightmare began at the very bottom of the stairs. The attacker, in her nightmare, wasn't himself, but a big, monstrous creature blocking her way up the stairs and out of the station. It wasn't until Lexi started engaging in healing work and, specifically, more embodied sex that she made progress on the dream. During acupuncture one time, she had the nightmare while in a half-waking state, and that small amount of consciousness allowed her to alter the dream, change the situation, and tell her nightmare assailant that he had no power in the situation. She walked out of the nightmare having resolved the situation, and never had the dream again.

In her waking life, Lexi engages in sex that isn't necessarily what outsiders would expect of a sexual assault survivor. With her current partner, Lexi has explored many dark, more intense sexual scenes, planned out carefully, including some elements of CNC. These stem from Lexi's desire to reenact aspects of sexual assault in a way she has control over, because she can say "stop" at any time. She comes up with scenarios she wants to play out, and discusses them at length with her partner, including safety measures and ways to pause or stop. Sometimes, the scenes can be "too spicy"—involving weapons, for example—and Lexi has had to keep some of these scenes off of her OnlyFans.

While many people might think CNC is more likely to trigger a trauma survivor, Lexi explains that a knife or a gun appearing in sex or in porn has never been a trigger for her. When those weapons come up, she expects it. It feels like exposure therapy. A big part of these scenes is building that feeling of safety in Lexi's body. Experiences that feel out of control, and activating to her nervous system, are rewired through her play to actually feel very safe. She is reprogramming her body to understand that she can be safe in the environment or context in which she was once in danger. What actually triggers her is usually something that surprises her. Vanilla sex, or brief sexual encounters, can trigger her, because there isn't the same context built up the way there is in a planned scene, even if it's more intense. Many survivors I spoke to touched on this idea: what makes sex feel safe is actually talking through what we want (our fantasies) before we get naked, not the particular type of sex we engage in.

Some of our fantasies originate before we were assaulted—and trauma can completely shift how we view those same fantasies later. Since adolescence, Matthew had the idea that if he slept with his imagined physical ideal partner—"lean, fairy, toned, tall"—then he would love the experience no matter what. But his whole concept of his ideal partner disintegrated when a person with that exact description assaulted him. "Looking back now, I had been chasing this idea of something that never really existed and still really doesn't," Matthew says. A person with any physical description can be a perpetrator, and sleeping with a certain kind of body type doesn't protect us from assaults. Matthew experienced a mismatch when it came to his aesthetic expectations and reality. Matthew also has found that sleeping with other people with his "ideal" body hasn't led to particularly great sex, either. For him, sex has become less about the aesthetic match and more about communication. He was influenced by porn and fantasies he'd had since he was much younger, and he had trouble letting go of those outside influences and homing in on what actually turned him on, not just checked a box. For Matthew, that exploration had to happen through trial and error in real life, and proved to be the opposite of his fantasy. Sometimes, trauma changes our inherited or cultural narratives around what we should fantasize about and gives us space to consider what we actually desire.

To Alisa, not all post-assault fantasies are what they appear at surface level. Sometimes, she's engaged in fantasy and role-playing that others might say is shameful or harmful. But those fantasies, acted out or just inside her head, make her feel embodied and powerful. She thinks it depends on the person to figure out what feels good to them. She explains, "I've been shamed for not having any sex. I've been shamed for having too much sex." If she can't win, Alisa feels she might as well do what feels good. What other people think can't be the metric by which we live our sex lives.

Alisa believes that our fantasies aren't just a reflection of our trauma, but it can be part of our healing. It's not about the type of sex you fantasize about or even engage in, she explains to me, because we can be making sexual choices "that are more reflective of our hurt, or . . . for reasons that are more reflective of us experimenting with our healing." She believes it's not about the kind of sex we're into—kink or vanilla, long-term monogamy or one-night stands—but rather "why we're making the choices we're making, and how it feels in our bodies." She follows one rule: If a fantasy feels healing to her, then it is. Sometimes, harnessing your imagination can be a helpful way of exploring how a new type of sex might feel, and playing inside your own head can be a more comfortable way to experiment before involving a partner.

Fantasies can be useful not only before or instead of having sex with a partner, but during, too. Leanna doesn't like to use restraints during sex. But if she wants to try something involving restraints, she ties them to a specific fantasy she can get her brain to latch onto, in case she panics. That way, the panic becomes part of the narrative around why she's consenting to the restraint. She tells herself, "This is what we're doing, why we're doing this."

Sometimes, Leanna's husband shows up to sex with a specific fantasy for the encounter that she didn't expect. If he doesn't mention his fantasy until after they get going, she sometimes has a negative reaction, like a panic attack. She wants to be prepared in advance and discuss it before they get started. Many survivors agree that they want partners to explicitly ask before trying new things—even survivors who are less into verbal, affirmative consent in general. Talking through a fantasy before engaging in it is a crucial way to keep everybody feeling safe.

Danika finds fantasy an effective way for her to process trauma—and orgasm. Sometimes to get out of her head, to feel safe enough to feel vulnerable during sex, she has to check out and go somewhere else. For Danika in particular, fantasy is an effective way of processing trauma and reflecting back the kind of relationships and sex we want in our real lives, because she is a romance writer. Danika writes romance as a way to process her sex life as well as her assaults. She sees it as healing, an exercise in imagination. She likes romance as a genre because either the negative part of the story is already over—it's the backstory—or it doesn't have to happen because the relationship is healthy. She is writing the world as she wishes relationships existed in it.

At an earlier point in her career, Danika worked on darker material. These days she's into "the healthy relationship, the communication, the no shame." She gains control of the narrative by writing the narrative. Writing, for Danika, is both a creative release and a way of envisioning healthy options for her future and her present. It's a more edited version of what many survivors do: we think before we act.

Leanna has been reading erotica since she was a young teenager, and has always found it a safe haven to explore sexually. After her trauma, she felt like retreating into erotica was a more comfortable way to continue developing her sexuality and self-pleasure. To her it felt safer, but still stimulating. She could skim over parts that weren't appealing to her, or things that made her feel nervous. It was a much more self-directed experience than porn, which felt difficult to control once it started. "As someone with trauma," Leanna explains, "you can interpret it your own way." She can "erase" parts of read material from her mind more easily than visual porn.

To me, porn feels out of control because I don't know what's coming next. That surprise factor is a turnoff for me. Similarly, I find that the first time I sleep with someone, when I don't know what they'll want to do next, I'm much more nervous. Once we've slept together, I become less anxious. Watching porn feels like signing up to be surprised, and potentially triggered, constantly. Other survivors put effort into finding and getting used to porn they enjoy, like Leanna, who puts work into picking nontriggering porn content through keyword searches and blocking upsetting categories, like heavily dom/sub dynamics, rape fantasies, and restraints. She treats it like one of the challenges of living with C-PTSD. Leanna is grateful she has explored with porn as a trial for real life experience.

Leanna finds that media depictions of violence or gore have put her off most movies and TV. Scenes of domestic violence or images of wounds from trauma bother her for obvious reasons, but Leanna is also bothered by content that resembles aspects of her trauma but isn't necessarily "violent." If there's a lot of tension, like during a psychological thriller, Leanna notices her panic response start to take hold. I have a similar reaction to gory or suspenseful video or visual content. I find it activates PTSD symptoms that were long dormant, especially hyperarousal or dissociation—my brain trying to protect me from a projected, alternate reality. Leanna, who experiences violent urges as a symptom of PTSD, sometimes feels that desire to act violently even if the threat is only present in a movie she's watching. Watching characters' reactions to trauma, like PTSD symptoms, also feels invalidating to Leanna. TV shows might turn something lifelong and complex into a two-episode plot device.

It isn't really possible to have a trigger warning for everything, since many people experience PTSD symptoms as a result of circumstance-specific triggers—for me, anything involving grabbing wrists or certain songs may make me panic. Most people wouldn't expect those to be triggering, but would expect other things to trigger me that don't—like being submissive to large men, or having sex with strangers. Since there's effectively no comprehensive trigger warning system, consuming media, from movies to erotica to porn, will always be difficult. But for many survivors, it's safer to imagine a sexual scene as part of self-pleasure than to watch unpredictable porn, or at least something that hasn't been screened first.

In the same vein as Leanna's reorientation around visual media, Alisa believes once we decide to share our fantasies and internal experiences, we have to be mindful of how we might impact our partner. Consent, to Alisa, plays into how fantasies may be helpful to our healing processes. You have to get consent from your partner before describing a fantasy that might be triggering. It's important for people to feel comfortable pumping the brakes on a conversation or the level of detail in a description. Sometimes she isn't in the right headspace to hear vivid descriptions of the harm, or descriptions of the flashback of the harm that's happening. This can even extend to describing triggers.

During conversations with new partners, Alisa explains that she wants "to hear about your experience being triggered and what you need in terms of support," but not the details of what happened—where the trigger originated. She believes our conversations about triggers and desire should be consent-based too. Navigating these conversations as directly as possible can help, as well as being intentional about the space you're building together.

Mason also plays with the border between fantasy and reality in order to be comfortable during sex. He uses imagined scenes to maneuver around his trauma-related discomfort. To receive pleasure, like oral sex, Mason needs to have something else going on in his head. If he's solely focused on his physical experience in the moment, it's hard to be present, and that can turn into a problem. When the focus is just on him, he finds it difficult to be present in his body in the room. Being the sole recipient of pleasure brings up feelings of unworthiness, and makes him feel like he immediately owes his sexual partner reciprocation. He has a hard time when he sees the pleasure as one-sided, even just while it's happening—a sentiment shared by many sexual assault survivors, especially around oral sex. Ignacio says receiving oral sex as a survivor is rough—not just for them. It involves a lot of vulnerability and can feel like too much emotional pressure. They usually avoid oral sex to completion so that they don't get stuck in their head and "float away." Mason has a similar reaction and opts to enter a different mental scenario, like a fantasy or an alternate storyline. That way, he's not completely in the room with his partner. When he fantasizes in these moments, there's always another person in the fantasy who is receiving pleasure alongside him. To Mason, the impact of the fantasy is what's most important, not necessarily the specific details of what's going on in his head. Mason doesn't see this as dissociation in the medical sense, since he's checking into controlled sexual fantasies, not just checking out mentally.

While this system technically works for Mason, he feels "deeply uncomfortable" with it. He wants to be more present during hookups, and he's gotten feedback from partners that they wish he could be more open to receiving pleasure from them. I also struggle to receive oral sex, and hearing from other survivors who felt similarly reassured me. It's confusing in a sexual climate where women are often advocating for their right to oral sex, even claiming that men who won't go down on them are bad sexual partners, and I'm actually running away from it—sometimes I wonder, what's wrong with me? But like Mason, I'm learning to stay within my own experience: I'm allowed to want what I want, and not want what I don't want. Today, Mason is working on mindfulness techniques to help retrain his brain. He's also found his current girlfriend to be helpful to this process, because he feels comfortable speaking openly about the issue with her. Keeping it all in his head has historically been a big part of the problem.

Mason believes it's important to talk to current partners about fantasies, including those involving previous lovers—those lines of communication should be open. He says, "Tell me all your dirty shit you've done before, I want to know it all." Understanding his partners' full sexualities helps him reach a more open level of communication about sex, and the relationship in general.

In talking to survivors, I noticed a theme: We have to practice radical acceptance of both trauma symptoms, like nightmares and panic, that may persist for years, and also acceptance of our desires and fantasies. We may like imagining scenarios that aren't what we think we "should" like—or we may find we actually don't like exploring our fantasies in real life. We may even be surprised to find we like what somebody else suggests in the heat of the moment. When partners have asked to try new desires, I've always learned a lot about my own sexual interests, even if all we do with a fantasy is talk about it.

Sharing the root of our fantasies, like sharing details of trauma, doesn't necessarily go well. Sometimes what I fantasize about feels just as out of control as a flashback. I often find myself attracted to men who look similar to the man who raped me when I was a teenager—long curly hair, beard, speaks another language natively. It is subconscious, just something I am drawn to. But the few times I've described where my attraction for somebody came from, people became defensive, not understanding that what turned me on was baked into my sexuality and part of who I am.

What we fantasize about and what reminds us of trauma can both have complicated roots. Understanding the origins of our desires and fears will only help us as we begin to seek out sexual experiences. An understanding of our internal landscape gives us a more grounded place from which to have conversations with potential and current partners about how trauma impacts sex—even when those conversations get heavy. Being comfortable sharing our stories is something we learn from practice—and from other survivors.

CHAPTER 5

To Tell or Not to Tell

B EFORE I WROTE this book, I wrote articles and essays about sexual assault, including about my own experiences. Doing this aligned with my values to help other survivors and to express my pain through art, but it posed a problem: Anybody who Googled my name would immediately learn traumatic details I might not choose to share with someone I was casually dating, or a partner I preferred to become close to on my own timeline.

The first person I dated seriously after my stories became available on the internet was Leo. We had briefly met years before, and he had followed my journey as a writer on social media since then. By the time we met again in real life, he had read everything I had ever published. Leo never questioned my narrative or asked me for details beyond what I was open to sharing in the moment, and he turned a potential opportunity for discomfort—him knowing more than I chose to tell him—into a strategy to listen more effectively. His familiarity with my trauma history gave us a shared lexicon to become physically and emotionally intimate. With other partners, disclosing my trauma history wasn't as all-or-nothing, and rarely did it have such positive results.

One of the topics survivors struggle with is whether or not—or if so, how—to share our trauma histories to people we choose to be intimate with. Some survivors use the term "disclosure" to describe the experience of sharing details of our trauma history, how somebody might disclose medical or financial information. But another form of disclosure I've experienced took place during the interviews I did for this book. In every interview, a survivor chose to share something difficult with me and that formed a connection between us. What they said resonated. Disclosure to a potential partner should have the same effect: to start a connected conversation.

Ignacio tells me that we begin to heal by sharing our stories. Disclosure of our trauma history is one form of that storytelling. They see it as a chain: "One person speaks, and that gives another person agency or permission to speak about something they didn't think they could." Ignacio sees our conversation as a form of normalization—just like my mission for the book as a whole. Communication allows more people to feel more connected, and less isolated. Ignacio wants to lend their "voice to the collective," and as they speak, I think to myself: That's what we want disclosure to sound like, too.

Stacey was a second responder for sexual assault survivors, meaning she supported them after the initial emergency when they came home from the hospital or from reporting to the police, or even later, if they needed logistical support with something like housing. In those moments, Stacey chose not to put aside her own lived experience, but to make use of her empathy. "That means not asking a ton of questions and being invasive or telling them what to do," Stacey explains, saying that they need to feel in control in those moments—at least of their social interaction, even if their life feels out of control. She knows, having been in their shoes, that how somebody reacts to your lived experience of trauma is something you never forget. She explained, up front, that if they want to tell her anything, that's fine, and if they don't, that's also fine. That way, the survivors would never have to question her role and what she wanted from them. She explained that they could tell her what they needed and she would figure out how to meet those needs. Stacey wishes she had had a second responder to help her, and thinks having a listening ear may have shortened the duration of her healing process. She knows that even if later responses to some-body's trauma disclosure are kind and positive, early responses hold a lot of weight and remain significant. She knows that while at the time she felt like a random person to survivors she was assigned to help, to them, it often had a more impactful meaning. Stacey's experience as a second responder informed what she later wanted out of partners' reactions.

One day, Stacey hopes to provide education for partners of sur-vivors on what they can do to be genuine pillars of support. She has observed many partners trying to make the situation revolve around their feelings and needs instead of the survivor's. Her past partners have reacted with self-centered questions: How will this affect me? How can I get more information about what happened to the survi-vor? They want to get to a more comfortable place in the conversation, but they center themselves when it would be more kind and more productive to shift the focus back to the survivor. That's what creates open lines of communication, she says, as well as the space to talk about how it's affecting both of you.

Stacey sees it this way: someone who has experienced trauma has fallen into a hole. They are looking for a partner to reach down into that hole and lift them up. Often, all the partner is talking to them about is: how did they fall down into the hole? How deep is the hole? They're asking about the hole, suggesting the survivor had actually walked in a different direction, and maybe they weren't in the hole at all. But the survivor in that moment of experiencing trauma really just needs the hand to pull them up—not the line of questioning about the trauma itself, which is all too common.

Looking back, Stacey wished she could have had better, clearer communication with her partner about her trauma history. If she could go back in time, she would tell him that trauma is like shattered glass: "When you drop a glass in your kitchen, you'll pick up all these pieces, but a year later you'll find a shard somewhere, and it is still very sharp. And you're still experiencing that same kind of pain when you find it, in all these unexpected places. You thought you cleaned

it all up—you're good to go—and then you're getting hurt again."
Her partner had to navigate those shards of glass with her without
knowing what they represented, and she wishes she could have given
him a better map. But she didn't have it before she had it, and now
she's happy that he's the person that will navigate her trauma with her
moving forward.

Bad responses to trauma can have a huge impact on how we move
forward. For me, some early negative reactions—disbelief, minimizing, and rejection—to my trauma had a negative impact on me, and
I withheld information from people who might have helped me for
years. A family member told me, "I knew something like this would
happen to you," and in that moment I felt more alone than I had since
the assault. You can never know how bad others' reactions will be
before you disclose to them. Choosing who to tell and who not to tell
is difficult, and ultimately, we can't control other people's reactions.

"Oversharing" and "trauma bonding" are discouraged by today's culture, but people using those terms are probably not referring to talking
about trauma as it relates to sex. Talking about the impact of trauma
on sex, especially with the people we sleep with, helps us have healthy,
safe, and pleasurable sex.

Lyndsey, the sex therapist, doesn't think there's one right way to
tell your partner about trauma. But she almost always recommends
disclosing. If somebody's partner isn't a safe person, or there's a specific reason a survivor won't talk to them, she recommends reflecting
on that reason and why they are with somebody with whom they
feel uncomfortable sharing. Sometimes in long-term partnerships or
marriages, a sexual dynamic can be difficult to navigate or lacking in
consent, leaving one partner feeling scared or violated and certainly
unwilling to open up about past trauma. In those cases, the priority
has to be safety, not sex or improving a couple's sex life by talking
about past trauma. The classic advice to schedule sex once a week can
be hugely harmful if one partner doesn't feel safe, or safe to lay down
boundaries or to say "no." If a conversation "risks retaliation," it is not

safe enough to speak, but if a safe space can be created, it can be worth addressing. Ultimately, Lyndsey believes it's up to the individual to decide whether or not to disclose.

If a survivor does want to disclose, Lyndsey suggests setting the intention to be to connect with them over their past. Some survivors question the premise of the conversation: what's the point? Lyndsey says disclosing gives your partner a chance to support you and for you to be vulnerable with them. She suggests explaining what happened by framing the conversation and the explanation of what happened to you as a way of getting to know each other better, and understanding what you've been through. You don't need to get into the nitty-gritty details of the trauma for the conversation to be impactful on the relationship. Disclosing the existence of trauma and the fact that it impacts the relationship can be a positive first step (or only step). Lyndsey has always expected the conversation to make her feel closer to her partner, but in reality, these conversations can have a wide array of outcomes, including negative ones. It's not in your control how somebody else reacts, though, and many survivors find it is worth disclosing regardless of how a partner responds.

In terms of timing a trauma disclosure, Lyndsey feels that in general, the earlier the better. Maybe not the first date, but before getting intimate with somebody. It also depends on an individual's journey: If we're talking about a recent trauma and it's still impactful, still causing triggers, disclosing early makes sense. If something happened twenty years ago, and the impact on sex and relationships is minimal, it may not be a high priority to disclose early. Or other personal information may be more important to focus on sharing, like relationship history or family issues. Lyndsey points out that if you sleep with someone and disclose the information only after, they could respond badly and make you realize they're not a "safe" person. Disclosing later on can be more harmful than starting the conversation early. It's okay to hold potential partners to the standard of whether they can have a healthy conversation about trauma—it's okay for that to be a primary criteria for choosing a partner. It may feel bad that something related to trauma can strongly influence your choice of who to date, but realistically, if you need a partner who is good at dealing with trauma, it's important to be clear about that not only with them, but with yourself, too.

Again and again, trauma survivors have expressed discomfort or unease about the idea of teaching their partners how to respond to trauma, or deal with symptoms of PTSD, or navigate conversations that may come up. I felt this way about early partners: Why should I have to do that extra work of educating somebody? In the end, I think it's a balance. A partner should have a foundational kindness and openness that predisposes them to having conversations with me that feel safe. I want to feel held. But at the same time, it's okay for me to teach partners how to respond to trauma. Everybody learns from someone. As I get older, and my partners get older, I find I'm usually not the first person they've dated or slept with who's experienced sexual trauma anymore, and I don't have to give that "introductory" conversation much. When I do, it still might feel frustrating or invalidating, but if I like someone enough and they are open to learning, I know that sharing what kind of response would be helpful to me will actually improve the experience for me, not just them.

For a living, Stacey gives talks about consent, sex, and sexual violence. Compared to work, she tells fewer people in her personal life the details of her trauma history. Audience members during a speech are people she's probably never going to see again. She'll talk to them personally, one-on-one, after her speeches, and she cherishes these interactions. They might talk about someone's specific experience, or more generally about systemic problems that played into those experiences. But she rarely sees those audience members again, so the conversations feel contained.

But one-on-one, with a partner or loved one, it's different. It's more raw, and leaves her feeling exposed. She's thought a lot about why she feels more open to having those one-on-one conversations with strangers. If it's somebody she knows personally, she's already invested in the relationship. She wants to continue the relationship with them, or maintain what they have. Once she discloses her trauma history, they're going to react. That person can't take back their reaction, and if it's not a positive one, it changes Stacey's relationship with them forever. That reaction can disrupt an otherwise positive long-standing relationship. It's why other survivors, like Lyndsey, believe in disclosing early with new people, to avoid that potential for a delayed negative reaction. Without an empathetic response, Stacey knows disclosing can have high stakes—even meaning the end of a relationship. The interaction might mean she loses control over how they see her and the relationship. "What if they don't believe you?" she explains. Being vulnerable is difficult, and if she regrets being vulnerable, that regret compounds on top of the trauma.

Stacey knows that telling people about her trauma directly is better than them finding out from a third party, pointing to research that suggests people are more likely to believe sexual violence occurred if they hear directly from the victim, and not secondhand (when they're likely to think it's false reporting).[1] She navigates these stakes constantly as a survivor of sexual assault who works publicly in this area.

Stacey's current, long-time partner has always made pointed jokes making fun of rape culture and how ridiculous some related opinions are. Those jokes show Stacey he has empathy and offers a safe space for Stacey to start conversations with him about her own life.

Before Stacey disclosed her trauma history to her current, long-term partner, she knew he could tell something was wrong. It wasn't always sexual triggers that came up, and she felt she couldn't explain those moments. Sometimes, a particular laugh would set her off, an audio trigger other people didn't notice. But she hadn't equipped her partner with the knowledge or tools to be supportive of her needs. She explains, "It's like someone who's uncomfortable with cats picking them up, and they're like . . . they wanna be nice to it but they don't know how to do it." Stacey felt like her boyfriend wanted to treat her with care, but without direction he kept fumbling it.

Three years into their relationship, after a triggering incident at home, Stacey told her long-term current partner to give her space.

She didn't want to talk, so he headed back to his place. A blizzard shut down work, so she stayed in and curled up watching the Lifetime TV series *Surviving R. Kelly*. She binged the whole show. Watching so many survivors be vulnerable and share their experiences prompted her to open up to the idea of sharing more of her story to her partner. Later that evening, she got on the phone with her partner to talk through the trigger, without intending to name its source—her past protocol in these situations. Instead of that usual approach—tiptoeing around the issue—she started talking about what she'd been up to that day, and the show came up.

"I think it's something you should watch," she remembers telling him, "I think it would help you understand why I behave the way that I do." She felt her shoulders tense throughout the conversation and, perhaps worried he wouldn't want to watch a whole TV show to understand her "meltdown," as she describes it, she pointed to one particular scene where R. Kelly's ex-wife ended up on a website that listed off the signs of sexual abuse. The ex-wife realized it described her experience. Stacey told her partner about the website, and reiterated that she was having the same experience as the ex-wife. She felt foolish, speaking in this roundabout way, having worked in sexual violence prevention for years, but long ago she had separated her work from her personal life, a necessary compartmentalization to get her through years of survival. She hoped her partner would receive the message she was trying to send.

Her partner didn't have the same professional background as her, or her understanding of what might be going on. So she used the TV show as a jumping-off point and explained that the website had more resources he could look at. He listened to her talk on the phone, taking in the information, absorbing what she was ready to share.

That conversation about a Lifetime TV show proved to be a turning point in their relationship. Stacey stopped feeling like she needed her partner to leave for her to calm down if she was triggered because now, he had a grasp on what was going on. The TV show reference gave them a shared language they could both use in later conversations. Before that conversation, she hadn't given him the information or had the conversations that might have enabled him to respond appropriately. By talking about her experience in the context of other survivors' experiences, she effectively normalized what happened to her while explaining her individual experience more clearly. This isn't a strategy specific to Stacey (or R. Kelly). Other survivors have used the #MeToo movement, a news cycle, or other pop culture references as a gateway into a more personal conversation. I've heard from survivors who used articles I've written about sex or rape to talk about what happened to them with their partner.

Other survivors take a different approach. Ramona says she tends "to be very upfront with people as fast as possible." She is wary of sharing details of trauma experiences, but even on a first date she'll ask clearly about the other person's goals for dating and what works for them in a relationship. She doesn't need to hear potential partners debate whether they're good matches for her, given her trauma history. She can consider that question on her own. Talking about serious stuff early paves the way for Ramona to commit to relationships that serve her needs.

A few dates in, Ramona tries to have honest conversations about how her trauma affects dating. Last summer, she went on two dates with someone. "We hit it off pretty well—we were messaging back and forth," Ramona says. She didn't like that he was on the clingier side (his words, not hers), but he felt right enough that she wanted to give it a chance. On their first date, they made out more than she was used to and he was handsy, but they had talked a lot about her sexual boundaries and she felt comfortable with their hookup on the whole.

On their second date, he groped Ramona repeatedly, and put his hands under her clothes without asking. It wasn't a clear-cut sexual assault experience to her, but it reminded her very clearly of times she had felt violated. She felt frustrated because of how easy it is to simply ask if it's okay to escalate an encounter, or to try a specific sex act. She felt he jumped way too quickly to something that wasn't in her comfort zone. Plus, his actions felt very different from how he had acted on the first date, and she was disappointed that he turned out to be so bad with boundaries. He apologized, and she felt it wasn't malicious, but they didn't go out again.

Ramona feels comfortable asking specific questions about the future to gauge how the other person feels so she can approach the relationship from a more stable place. Early on, she asked her current boyfriend if he wanted to get married, have kids, and have a certain amount or kind of sex. They originally met on OkCupid but didn't feel any chemistry at the time, though they became friends and even collaborated on work projects. Ramona became interested in pursuing a romantic relationship, partly because she felt she'd done enough "research" on him to feel comfortable with sharing trauma.

Many survivors put disclosing trauma in the same general category as coming out. Ramona lists "asexual" in her dating app profile bios, and tries to get into more specifics about what that means for her, too. "Most people's impression of asexuality," Ramona explains, "is, 'Oh, that means you don't want to have sex with anyone ever.'" That doesn't match Ramona's experience of asexuality. She usually says, "I enjoy having sex with partners I'm serious with." Ramona has noticed an "infantilization that comes with [asexuality], and an assumption that you don't know anything about sex." In tandem with feeling like she has to do the work of explaining her trauma history, Ramona feels like dating can require a lot of vulnerability.

Mason is bisexual and has dated mostly women. When he has disclosed his trauma history in the past, usually in tandem with his coming out as bi, most of the women he's dated had a very passive response and seemed more concerned about what this meant for them than what it meant for him. They would be like, "Oh cool," but, in Mason's words, "You could tell that a lot of them were not very cool with it." He noticed it emasculated him in their eyes, or it worried them. Sometimes they would barely respond beyond that initial acknowledgment, moving the conversation on to something else—what they would do for dinner. Some of them would respond with curiosity, but Mason believes their questions were usually about assuaging their own insecurities about his masculinity or because what he said made them feel bad. Some of them made his bisexuality into a new reason to be jealous of his other relationships.

Disclosing his early sexual assaults alongside his bisexuality was mostly a negative experience until his most recent relationship with his current girlfriend. About his bisexuality, she responded, "Oh— hot," and opened up the conversation for him to discuss his past and self. She made him feel loved in that conversation, which was "mind-blowing" for Mason.

Even with friends, Mason has struggled to explain his trauma history and bisexuality, which he sees as part of the same conversation. Some of them have assumed Mason was sharing his story because he was into them. Mason doesn't see friends sexually, and gay and bi men "exist in a completely different category in my mind." All these negative and unhelpful responses have left Mason feeling like it's hard to be his full, authentic self. He always has on a mask.

Mason remembers telling a woman he was seeing about his trauma history and bisexuality. Mason regretted telling her immediately—he could see in her body language and verbal reaction that she wasn't going to stick around. Though they kept seeing each other for a couple of more months, she refused to have sex with him again. It was disappointing for Mason that she, "a young, white, liberal woman" couldn't be open and accepting of his past in an actual intimate relationship. She completely failed to meet his needs. She had even shared some of her own trauma history with him, but she failed to see him as somebody who had also been hurt and deserved just as much support as she did. When both partners have experienced trauma, balancing each other's needs and respecting each other's boundaries is important—no different than the needs or boundaries of a partner that hasn't experienced trauma, but handled with a little extra sensitivity. Mason has had some version of that interaction with every woman he has seriously dated.

When Mason considers when to tell new partners about his trauma history, he is wary of sharing too much up front. But he doesn't want to get to a place where he feels like he's hiding important parts of himself from somebody he's starting to care about—or to have someone accuse him of withholding information. Ultimately, Mason makes the call to share his history if hiding it means outright lying about who he is, or if a conversation would go differently if they knew—even if it's joking about if Timothée Chalamet is hot or not. "The straight act has to drop in order for there to be a further, deeper level of conversation, or intimacy," Mason says.

Mason discloses by telling somebody he is bi first, and then, more often than not, he ends up talking about how he connects that to his early childhood sexual trauma. Mason faces a lot of stigma over his bisexuality, and the added layer of trauma disclosure makes open conversations even more difficult. But he feels the context of his traumatic experiences rounds out the explanation of his sexuality in a way that feels most whole.

Mason hasn't been in a serious relationship with a man, and he finds he doesn't feel the need to disclose his trauma history with casual hookups. Mason hasn't ever been with a man to the extent that he feels it would be appropriate to disclose trauma. He doesn't think disclosing his sexuality or what he calls the "backstory" (his trauma) is appropriate for something short-term. It's "at least third or fourth date stuff." The only conversation about his trauma history Mason has had with a man was with his best friend—he's the only man Mason has told the whole story to. That kind of friend can feel extra valuable.

Lexi joined a women's circle after deciding to get serious about her healing journey. Early on, some other members of the women's circle invited her to visit the hot springs, naked. Lexi said no—for two years. When she finally did join them, she wore a bikini. The next time, she wore just the bottoms. Eventually, she joined the group of women nude.

A couple of weeks before we spoke, Lexi went back to the hot springs and undressed. Forty-five minutes into the visit, she realized she hadn't had a single thought about her body since she arrived. The other women there had witnessed her in all her different healing phases, in all her different sizes throughout her journey. Lexi believes that those women witnessing her as she changed was where her healing came from. "The idea that we have to be healed before we can be in real connection with people, I find so harmful," Lexi says, "because I think so much of the really impactful healing that we do happens in community with other people. We don't do it alone. We were never meant to do it alone." Sharing yourself and being open about how you heal and grow is part of how you get better—you can't show up fully healed, you have to get there together.

Lexi says, "It's almost like there's this incentive to hide who you are and what you're actually feeling, because you're supposed to be healed." That can lead to serious issues when you're already struggling to communicate your needs and what's happening in your body and mind during sex. Lexi describes the "container of the relationship" where healing can actually take place in the most impactful way. It's all about, in Lexi's words, "showing up vulnerably and honestly and with the intention of connection." To her, conversations about trauma history and how trauma continues to show up are part of connecting.

Lexi points out that even if you do a ton of healing work before having any kind of sexual relationship or body-based interaction post-assault, new stuff will probably come up in your first relationship, even if it's the same relationship from before the assault. New activities, new contexts, and changes to the relationship can bring up issues that you would never have encountered while trying to heal alone.

By the time she met her husband, Leanna had a "canned answer" to describe the trauma she had endured. "I think this is the case for a lot of people where you just come up with this reporter-style summary, and it's very objective. It's very distanced." When she talks about the trauma itself, it feels like she's talking about somebody else as the victim. She sees it as a form of dissociation, but I have heard other people describe the same phenomenon as a form of protecting yourself emotionally. "It's a way to explain without necessarily identifying with it." Leanna leaves out details of the assault when she gives this summary, like how she got away, or how far the assault went. Some of those details might come later, in a relationship with more built trust. That initial brief summary was what Leanna gave her husband the first time she disclosed her trauma history to him.

I find friends feel much closer after I've shared some aspect of trauma history. While this feels positive in the moment, and sharing, in my experience, tends to be a good idea, it can lead to a false closeness that isn't necessarily earned. Trauma has made me lean into snap judgments—this person feels safe enough to be open with, that person I reject. Often, reality is somewhere in between, and sharing information shouldn't be a more important consideration than other aspects of a relationship, whether friendship or romantic.

Leanna didn't disclose her trauma history to her husband until the first time they were trying to have sex, mid-make out in the back seat of his car. "I panicked and burst into tears," Leanna says. He was confused—what was going on? She decided it was time to tell him. She thinks, looking back, that that panic attack was triggered less by the sex itself and more by some of the interpersonal aspects of their relationship she found triggering at the time: promising to spend time together and then having to cancel, for example. She didn't understand, back then, how much those circumstantial triggers escalated her nervous system leading up to sex. She was new to her own trauma and more used to the intense flashbacks or severe dissociation than a slow buildup of triggering situational factors.

Leanna suggested they climb from the back seat to the front and talk. She started crying, and he became upset, too, thinking something he had done had caused her distress. During that conversation he shared he was sad for her, and sorry for whatever he might have done to contribute to her reaction. Since then, "He's been absolutely brilliant at respecting boundaries, and stopping when I need him to or doing things a different way," Leanna says. She thinks her situation may differ from the norm because her husband was her first-ever long-term sexual partner. They learned to navigate her trauma together. After she told him her trauma history, he wanted to stay with her, be intimate with her, and join her in figuring out how to navigate a sexual relationship influenced by trauma.

Leanna felt like the focus with her husband was less on exploring her trauma narrative together and more on how it affected intimacy and boundaries. After they'd tackled those issues in their relationship together, the actual details of the trauma didn't seem that important. She thinks if she asked her partner today about which details he remembers, he would list a few, but that would be it. "I doubt he even thinks about it anymore," she says. I have had the same experience asking a long-term partner about a detail of my trauma I remember telling him, but he had completely forgotten about it. I wasn't mad, because he was always present in the relationship and worked on persisting triggers and issues, but it was jarring. I know other survivors might not feel as mildly about their partner forgetting traumatic details they've shared, even years later—it's up to the individual.

Leanna's husband accepted her trauma history completely the first time she shared it with him. She thinks this immediate receptivity— an unusual response, she recognizes—is "probably part of why I've been with him for so long." For trauma survivors, a partner's response to disclosure can be a prioritized criteria determining if we'll continue the relationship.

She remembers him telling her he wanted to help her with whatever she needed, and that he encouraged her to tell him when he was doing something wrong. She points out that the encouragement to point out (essentially, diagnose) what's wrong in the moment is actually a mixed message and difficult to enact. "You can't always articulate what's going on and when to tell someone to stop," Leanna says. She might freeze up or panic. Her mind starts "fighting with itself," trying to balance her actual needs in the moment with what her partner expects of her. She has to balance what she is afraid might be about to happen versus what is actually happening. Part of her brain tells her to "swallow it down," and part of her brain tells her to speak up. At the core of her internal struggle is her fear of jeopardizing the relationship.

I am a writer, and I've been sharing stories about myself, even about trauma, since before I had a driver's license. But those skills don't always translate to in-person conversations. I ask Danika if her career as a romance writer has had an impact on how she's navigated healing. "I am a person who communicates," Danika answers, "and it both reduces conflict and creates conflict." Danika shares how she's feeling during conversations, so those discussions dive deep. Sometimes in talk therapy, Danika notices how recognizing her emotions helps her regulate them. Outside her writing, Danika doesn't identify as a particularly good storyteller, and she's had a hard time talking about trauma.

When it came to disclosure to partners, Mia felt the topic came up naturally—it was 2018 in the United States, and rape was constantly in the news. She tells me she ended up disclosing her trauma history before she even knew if she was interested in people she was dating at that time. Her disclosure was somewhat surface level, though, and she shut down when a couple of people tried to dig deeper because she didn't feel she could explain further, since it was so early in the relationship.

Years after the rape, Mia rattled off the whole story to a newer friend, without using the word "rape." The new friend affirmed that what happened was by any definition rape. She called the attacker names, told Mia he was trash, and acted staunchly protective. While her friend's words aren't clear in Mia's memory, her face, reaction, and body language in the moment stick out. The fact that Mia still occasionally slept with the same man who raped her was distressing to her new friend. She remembers thinking that if this woman, who she'd known for no more than a few months, had such an extreme reaction, Mia had to reconsider her interpretation of what happened to her. That conversation led her to completely cut off contact with the attacker. This disclosure to a friend influenced Mia's thinking more than any conversation she would go on to have with future partners.

When Mia shared what happened to her with her mother, who is a trained therapist, "She reacted less like a therapist, and more like a mom." Mia appreciated her mom's response because, in her words, "I needed my mom." Her work as a therapist came into play, too. Mia recalls that her mom "also had the tools to actually talk to me about it, and figure it out." She thinks her mom's presence in her healing process helped her stay on track with her life, enabling her to start the school semester on time just a week later. But she didn't talk to her mom about it on an ongoing basis after that. Sometimes her mom brings it up as it relates to Mia's dating life—she might point out the assault could be causing problems with trust and self-worth, or making her feel "disposable," as Mia describes it. But she and her mom don't often have in-depth conversations about her trauma, unless it's causing problems.

After the assault, Mia slept with a few people to whom she didn't disclose her story because she didn't feel it was relevant, since they were so casual. Eventually she started dating somebody more seriously, and she told him about her trauma history a couple of months into their relationship. She tried to tell him about the assault as a bit—a joke—but he made her stop and have the full, real conversation with her: "'Run that back real quick,'" she remembers him saying. Mia thinks this disclosure affected how he treated her, but didn't necessarily impact how she approached their sex life. Today, Mia doesn't feel the trauma disrupts her day-to-day life. She has been in therapy for four years—with "an actual professional, not my mom."

Lexi sees the kind of slow, noticing-based healing that bodywork entails as a good model for practicing having difficult or vulnerable conversations, like when disclosing trauma to a partner. Start with a topic that doesn't matter as much to you, but shares similar characteristics to disclosing trauma, like sharing personal information or talking about something that happened in the past. Practice talking about something embarrassing or that brings up shame, or is unresolved from the past. Build the muscle slowly.

Getting diagnosed with autism and ADHD made Lexi aware that she is more honest and blunt than some of her peers. She isn't trying to change those qualities—they're just part of who she is. She has an agreement with her current partner when it comes to bringing a third into their relationship: "We're gonna show up as fully ourselves. And if we're not for you, we're not for you." Lexi feels less inherently threatened when sleeping with other women, but when she's playing with a new man, she might disclose her trauma history so they're on the same page. She'll say, "I have been sexually assaulted a myriad of times in my lifetime, and I have been very seriously assaulted." She then explains how that trauma manifests as triggers or challenges for her when it comes to sex. She tries to answer the questions, for herself and her partner: What are my limits? What are my triggers? What are my "fuck yeahs"? What are my "no's"? And, What are things we could potentially play with later on, but are "maybe's" for now?

Many survivors feel it's okay to hold off on disclosure until the right moment. Lexi points out that on top of the trauma of sexual assault, there can be a lot of self-inflicted pain and suffering after the traumatic event. We blame ourselves, or other people blame us when we open up with our stories. We can't control other people's reactions, but we can choose to be kind to ourselves, and process things in a way that doesn't completely overwhelm our nervous system all at once. That can mean waiting to have difficult conversations.

When she plays as a dom, Lexi prioritizes the same level of consent, based on honesty and awareness. "If you can't articulate your desires, limits, needs, concerns, triggers, any of that—if you don't feel comfortable to disclose the intimate details of it, that's totally fine," Lexi says. "But if you have an inability to articulate what's going on with you, and what your limits are, and how you feel, and what you're desiring—that's a hard pass for me as a dom playing with people," Lexi explains, continuing, "I need to feel safe that you, again around the consent issue but in reverse, like I need to trust that you will say no if something is a no." She needs to have enough trust with partners that if they feel bad, they'll speak up.

Lexi feels like there is no right or wrong way to disclose, and it's fine to not disclose at all in certain scenarios. But if a particular hookup requires trust, more disclosure feels important to Lexi. Quick, drunken vanilla hookups? Less necessary. Encounters involving power play or control? More important. She knows that her autism means she loves context to better understand how everything is working together around her. It just makes sense to her that more context is better, and helps her understand the nuance of an interaction. Plus, it allows her to hold the space her partner or partners need. She didn't learn to give all this context from some outside source, like sex ed or porn; this was something purely driven by her autism and her desire for context and information sharing. This style of communicating isn't limited to sex, but she finds it particularly helpful in establishing consent and trusting sexual relationships.

While Lexi and her partner agree that the male options they typically see on dating apps usually prove terrible at communicating, Lexi thinks the women they're talking to aren't actually much better at it—they're just held to much higher standards, so they have to improve. If women tend toward people pleasing, they'll end up communicating better not because they're inherently better at it, but because the world expects it of them.

Lexi has noticed that women and folks assigned female at birth (AFAB) often struggle to get diagnosed with autism for longer because they develop a people-pleasing, mask-building coping strategy that doesn't end up imposing on other people—which could trigger pressure to get a diagnosis—in the same way as male counterparts. Lexi's ability to hide her trauma similarly affected her ability to have relationships and bury trauma symptoms and the ways trauma impacts her experience of relationships. Masking, whether of autism or traumatic stress, served as a survival tool at certain points, but ultimately didn't help Lexi live in alignment with her values.

Having conversations about your trauma history starts the conversation of getting your needs met. It also helps build trust in and with your body—you're communicating to yourselves that you get to advocate for what you need, Lexi says. You deserve to be loved and held through difficult conversations, and you get to be with somebody who understands, because they have the context.

For Matthew, who hasn't had any long-term relationships in the years since his assault, there has never been quite "the right time or place to talk about that experience." While dating, he never felt like his trauma history came up organically, especially since he has primarily been on first or second dates, which he feels are not the right moment for a serious conversation. But Matthew's hesitation also came from an imposed message—don't talk about sexual assault in a romantic context, because nobody wants to hear about it (similar to Mason's experience dating). This is partly a reflection of Matthew's discomfort in hearing about somebody else's sexual assault on a first date. "If the interest is not mutual," Matthew says, "then it just becomes an uncomfortable topic." Matthew feels most comfortable discussing his assailant as an ex who "hurt him in a really serious way." He is wary that talking about sexual assault might be a turn off for someone who would otherwise be interested. He also feels that disclosing his trauma history might be a sign he is attaching to somebody more quickly than makes sense.

When it comes to hearing other people's stories, Matthew tries to be as empathetic as possible in case someone else is trying to broach the subject and finds it difficult, too. He also stays open-minded to letting others determine if the story they're telling is sexual assault or something else, always allowing each individual to make their own judgment about their own experience.

Matthew's approach is an intersection of wanting to listen and being hesitant to share his own story. Some people want to keep assault-related conversations to a minimum. There's a balance to be struck, and one guy I slept with did a great job maneuvering around my issues with his own boundaries. Aaron and I weren't compatible on every level, but both of us prioritized clear and direct communication. I knew he was fresh out of a breakup and feeling weighed down emotionally. He had told me he was only looking for a friends-with-benefits situation, and I was processing recent trauma and wasn't seriously dating, either. One night, when it became obvious that I was becoming anxious while we were making out, Aaron scooted a foot away and made eye contact with me. My body tensed, braced for a rejection due to my trauma.

"I'm not in a place to hear the details about what happened to you that's making you feel bad right now," Aaron said, "but I do want you to feel comfortable, so if there's anything I can do that would make you feel better, I'd love to hear it."

My whole body relaxed. The truth was, in that moment I didn't need to tell Aaron about any of the bad things that had happened to me. But I could use his help calming down. I asked him to tell me a story about his day, to ground me, and reached out to hold his hand. Aaron's redirection of my energy from disclosure to in-the-moment needs stabilized me—plus, it gave us the tools we both needed to move forward and have sex once I was calmer.

In an emotionally loaded moment during sex with a different man, I was asked point-blank why I was upset by a trigger. Unable to regulate my emotions in the moment, I chose to share the whole backstory behind the trigger. He became overwhelmed by the details and did not know how to react. I managed to guide us back to safer emotional ground, but the interaction spooked the guy and we did not see each other again. I blamed myself and the way I felt I had wrongly calculated how to handle the situation. Eventually, I considered that it takes two people to mishandle a situation, and maybe that man could be held accountable for asking prying questions during loaded moments.

Being able to set boundaries and tell difficult stories about our lives to a partner is important, but so is being able to receive boundaries (and trauma histories). Understanding what will make us feel comfortable in those conversations is crucial, because conversations with sexual partners go two ways.

A man I met on Tinder in my twenties asked to read something I wrote about the intersection of sex and trauma. I shared a piece I'd written for a women's magazine, a polished account edited down to some bare details—a piece of the puzzle, but not the whole picture. He responded compassionately and I decided to go out with him. When I later slept with him and had a panic attack, he reacted the complete opposite from the way I would expect somebody armed with the amount of information about me, and about sex and rape in general, would react. I spiraled into a panic attack so severe it lasted days. Sometimes, disclosing trauma doesn't yield a supportive reaction.

Alisa was honest with a partner about her history of CSA (childhood sexual abuse), and instead of being supportive, he accused her of not trusting him enough to sleep with him, the way a nontraumatized person could (according to him). Looking back, she sees his behavior as manipulative, but at the time it was difficult to see at twenty-two years old. His manipulation worked, and she believed she had to have sex with him to prove she trusted him. Halfway through sex, she realized she wanted to stop. She was letting her desire to prove him wrong override what her body was telling her she actually wanted. She got triggered, but even then her partner continued to accuse her of lying about her motives. He insisted this was really about her feelings towards him and ultimately left in the middle of the night.

Later, Alisa tried to sit down with him and have another, separate conversation to resolve the conflict that he had created. "He was the first guy I had given any indication to about what had happened, and I felt like I was put on trial," she shared. He insisted that if she had really been assaulted, she would know more about her own story, or have the particular reaction he imagined a survivor of assault would have—the myth of the perfect victim.

In retrospect, Alisa realized that a lot of her trust in him and belief in his good intentions stemmed from his job at a feminist organization, while his actual behavior toward her proved far from feminist, or even compassionate at a basic level. It can be difficult for trauma survivors to form healthy attachments with new people, either striving to become too close too fast or keeping unnecessary distance from people. Paying attention not only to the big picture—somebody's job, how they act when you first meet—is important, but so is keeping track of complicating factors and changing dynamics.

Alisa's first negative experience of disclosure haunted her for years. She had to unlearn all the false messages that guy pushed on her. Many survivors who have a bad experience of disclosure face the difficult task of unlearning the harmful messages they absorb from it. Alisa eventually realized her ex was approaching the interaction centering his own needs, when she needed her needs to be centered, or at least for them to share the spotlight. In her words, "everyone's boundaries matter." Alisa reflects, "People who make you feel like you are broken, like you are damaged goods, are not people you want in your life . . ." and continues, "We live in a world that likes to stigmatize us and tell us it's our fault—not just for what happened, but for the ways that we learn to survive, and the ways we learn to heal." Alisa's partner made her feel shame on every level.

One bad experience doesn't mean every disclosure going forward will be difficult, too. When Alisa met her husband, she started by telling him part of the story. She said, "I'm dealing with some trauma having to do with a parent, and they've shown up in nightmares that are kind of sexual." He reacted well and didn't press her. It was a full two years before she fully shared all the details. It wasn't about her partner; she wasn't being fully honest with anybody. He met her with "such love and such patience and such compassion that it just made it less scary" to tell him the full story when the time finally came.

When it comes to disclosure, Alisa believes that she, and all survivors, are "experts in our own safety and healing." It's up to us to decide how that will manifest when it comes to communicating about trauma. In her experience, that can look like anything from repressing traumas and pretending they never happened to "list[ing] my traumas out for you in alphabetical order, with a binder, with citations." But most of the time Alisa found herself somewhere in between. Ultimately, she finds comfort and empowerment in the idea that she gets to decide. She explains, "I don't have to have this profoundly logical reason why, with one sexual partner, I'm going to give a heads-up, and with another one, I'm not . . . it's enough that I'm trusting my own inner expert to help me navigate. And it doesn't mean that we can predict the future and we can control other people." Sometimes if Alisa believes a person feels safe for her to give a heads-up to, she might say, "I'm healing from some trauma, so it might show up. If I have a reaction to something, don't take it personally." She tries to provide at least a little context for any reaction she might have that might otherwise cause a partner to be confused or have an inappropriate reaction.

Lyndsey, like many survivors, has come to the realization that her list of must-haves in a partner can include being good at handling trauma. I, personally, had a hard time reconciling that fact, because I wanted my priorities to be based around who I was, not who I felt trauma had made me. But realistically, sexual and relationship goals change after sexual trauma. Being in touch with yourself enough to accept those changes is part of healing, and recognizing the importance of a partner who can work well with you around trauma helps set you up for success.

If a partner doesn't respond well, Lyndsey firmly believes everybody has the right to give them feedback, like, "The way you responded made me feel really bad and like I can't talk to you about this." She points out that a partner may have a bad response not because they don't care, but because they don't have experience or education in how to respond well. It can be helpful if a partner explains what led to their bad response. Some good questions Lyndsey thinks partners can ask include: What can I do? What do you need from me? Even if it's just the space to talk about the trauma. Sometimes a partner doesn't know what to do, and telling them can be helpful. Lyndsey says you can simply tell them, "When I say I need to stop, that means I need us to stop. I would like you to cuddle me, or maybe give me space—whatever works for you." It's important to say what you actually need in the moment to help mitigate the impact of trauma, de-escalate a panic attack, and feel better. This kind of direct communication is important because otherwise, they may do something that makes you feel worse.

If a partner digs their heels in and makes you feel bad for sharing that their response had a negative impact on you, that's probably not someone you want to be with. If you realize somebody is going to have a bad response to your trauma consistently, it makes sense to question whether that's even a person you want to be with. That isn't a safe space.

More than once in my life, I told somebody about my trauma history early, before I knew much about them. I prefer to see if a potential partner will have a bad reaction right away, so I don't waste my time. In a couple of cases, the partners I told about my trauma history held on to the knowledge I gave them for weeks. Then, during vulnerable moments, they each twisted what I said and tried to use it against me, to make me feel guilty and ashamed—to manipulate me. Telling is not always positive, and no matter how much you work to protect yourself from potential bad reactions, you might get one (and sometimes a delayed one).

When I've gotten those negative reactions, especially after a delay in which I felt I was actually building trust with somebody, I've felt deeply betrayed. The relationships were never able to recover, and I felt more closed and cut off than before I'd shared. In those cases, I've always ultimately ended contact with the potential partner. It made me feel gaslit, questioning my own reality, when somebody who seemed like they were on my side turns out to have been tricking me the whole time. Turning to friends and people you trust in those moments is crucial to mentally bouncing back. It may feel terrible in the moment, but if it's something you want, one day you'll end up with a partner who would never do that to you.

Not all survivors disclose their trauma histories—ever. Jennifer wrote me that she had never told her partner (now her husband) about her sexual assault. She didn't feel it was necessary for the relationship to function, because he was understanding and met her needs as is.

For many people, though, talking through our trauma histories is a challenge we have to face at least once. And for people who are single or dating at the time of our assault, it may feel like a necessary one. But that initial disclosure is only part of a much longer conversation. As your own relationship to your trauma history changes, your needs and wants related to sex may change, too, and keeping a partner in the loop is necessary.

After a string of casual encounters that left her emotionally exhausted, Gabby was ready for a relationship that felt safe and satisfying. "I realized that if I wanted to have loving sex, I would have to disclose [the assault] to my partner," Gabby explained. It wasn't as easy as a one-time disclosure. She realized the conversation had to be ongoing.

For a long time, Matthew needed somebody else to provide validation of his trauma and pain. It was helpful to him to have the same few friends available to talk about his experience over and over again. A few other people he spoke to about his trauma reproached him, saying "Are you seriously still talking about that?" Matthew reflects that that was "one of the hardest things to hear from people that you care about." He astutely describes the aftermath of his assault: "It's like this experience hasn't ended for me, and they don't necessarily get it." Talking about sexual assault and the impact of trauma is not a moment in time: it's an ongoing conversation. Even with the same partner, the conversation can change as you change as a person.

It's not just about talking about trauma or trauma symptoms—sometimes I want to talk about sexual encounters, and make sense of partners' reactions. One place I make space to talk about my sexual journey post-assault is not just with friends or longtime partners, but with new people I sleep with. I reflect on past sexual experiences by talking about past partners with people I'm currently sleeping with. I find that the intimacy I have with sexual partners creates space for more open-minded conversations—for growth. Talking about past partners might feel strange, but centering conversations like this on your personal experience of those encounters—whether it's sex or a conversation on a past first date—can make space for a safe conversation, both to process and to move forward in a more healthy way.

CHAPTER 6

First Times

THE FIRST SEXUAL trauma I remember experiencing as a kid would go on to affect me for my entire life, but at the time it happened, at ten years old, I did not have the contextual knowledge about sex or assault to understand why it felt bad. Those early assaults made me afraid of my own sexuality for many years, and I didn't start exploring until I had moved away from home and could break away from my old identity, rooted in trauma. Rather than sleeping with somebody in my friend group who I worried could gossip about my lack of experience, I chose a random guy in a bar to go home with when I was eighteen.

His name was Tomer, and at twenty-one years old, he felt miles beyond my maturity. He had just finished a few years in the army and his muscles, foreign beneath my fingertips, felt smooth as he drew me to him on his couch. I remember what I was wearing: a cobalt cotton skater dress from Urban Outfitters, worn-out flip-flops, and a touch of mascara. I cannot remember his face or voice, but I remember how my body lit up under his touch.

Most of my friends were losing their virginity to high school boyfriends or new college sweethearts—people they knew and trusted. I didn't plan to lose my virginity to Tomer—I was just tired, I think, of not being touched, or touching anybody else. I liked that there were no strings, that we would likely never see each other again, that we didn't have feelings for each other that might complicate things. Even then, during my first sexual experience, what mattered most to me was whether or not I felt in control.

Tomer took out a condom as he drew me to his bed. "I don't want to have sex like *that*," I said, not feeling confident enough to fully name my desire, but recognizing my boundary around intercourse.

"Just in case," he said, and placed it on the shelf by his bed. Years later, I would look back and recognize that what he did was a dismissal of a verbal boundary, but at the time I was glad he listened to me at all.

He lifted my dress and touched me—too much pressure, too fast a rhythm—but it thrilled me that I finally felt I had access to my sexuality. I enthusiastically took off my frayed Aerie bra and he pulled off my dress. He undid his belt and slid off his pants, and I scooted down to the edge of the bed. His penis tasted like skin—a surprise. He asked me to do something with his balls, and I got overwhelmed. Perhaps realizing I might have had less experience than he expected for somebody willing to have a one-night stand, he took over. Not long after, he came on my chest, handed me a paper towel, and ten minutes later I was on my way to my own bed. I felt proud, revved (later, I would recognize this just meant I hadn't come), and slightly sticky. When I told one of my roommates about the experience the next morning, I said "hooked up," and not understanding I had never slept with anybody, she assumed penetrative sex. I didn't correct her, because it very much felt like I had slept with him. Over the following years, my definition of sex would expand to include many more things than penetrative intercourse, and looking back, I always count this is as my first time.

After that first sexual experience with Tomer, I was freer about sleeping with people, making out with strangers, and generally tapping into my sexuality. Even dancing felt more flirtatious. It would be over a year before I had penetrative sex, because there was still a little voice in my head (a remnant of the purity culture I was steeped in, even growing up Jewish in liberal Massachusetts) that said the first penis that I let inside my vagina should be one attached to somebody

I knew well, and I wasn't seriously dating anybody. When, after I was raped, I did eventually meet the guy I would go on to date for years, David, I put off sex for months, afraid of the impact trauma might have on sex with him.

After we had penetrative sex for the first time, I was a little let down. It didn't feel life-changing, and all the reaction I had expected from my first time having penetrative sex just wasn't there. Sure, it was a slightly different physical sensation, but I'd already been intimate with David for months, and the feeling of pleasure remained the same. Lacking the emotional response I was supposed to feel, I put off telling friends for weeks. Many of these friends had thrust their own beliefs about virginity on me, and told me that just because I'd previously hooked up with somebody, I was still a virgin.

When I eventually told a friend about the sex I'd had with David (by then, we'd had sex multiple times), she asked me why I hadn't said anything since it was a big deal to lose your virginity. I shrugged, unsure how to explain myself. My definition of my "first sexual experience" had nothing to do with PIV (penis in vagina sex) and everything to do with the sexual awakening I'd experienced with Tomer. Plus, defining sex as something that requires a penis completely erases my bisexuality.

In truth, the real "big deal" I had felt having sex with David was all tied up in trauma. Unable to explain myself to my friend, I felt alienated, like something was wrong with me: I was supposed to care about my virginity. It wasn't normal to primarily care about how having sex related to being raped.

When something very bad happens to me, sexual trauma or otherwise, having sex for the first time feels more significant to me than "losing my virginity" ever has. And while some survivors I've spoken to don't share my perspective, most acknowledge that there are many more firsts that deserve our time and attention as we navigate sex and relationships.

Ramona was raised in a conservative Christian culture. "The idea of virginity was paramount," Ramona says. "It was the basis for every conversation about sexuality. It was the basis for how you relate physically, or don't relate physically, with someone, and how you enter marriage." She was baffled by the idea that sex went from being sinful to being a requirement on your wedding night, and then part of your everyday for the rest of your life. She received the message that masturbation was only okay if you masturbate thinking about your husband. Ramona only started masturbating a few years ago, and regrets that she didn't begin discovering sexuality as a child, how she perceives others to have done.

As an adult, Ramona landed on the other side of the virginity debate. "I just don't believe in virginity, just generally. I don't think that it's a real thing." Ramona thinks virginity is a concept made to control women. Just how women used to be predominantly treated like property, virginity was invented to give women a sense of value that could be tracked.

Ramona recalls her mom explaining what sex would be like the first time, including the assumption that she would break her hymen, bleed, and feel pain. Ramona reflects, "Maybe some people have that experience, but I don't think [when] you're having sex, you should be bleeding." She thinks this has to do with how people associate violence and sexuality, and pain and sexuality, with women. "It is assumed that women will go through pain as a result of sex," Ramona says, breaking down how virginity myths infiltrate our conception of sex throughout our life. She doesn't think that has to be true, and points out that we don't think of men's bodies in the same way.

Ramona doesn't buy into the idea that you have to "sleep with yourself" before having sex with somebody else. She thinks there's some truth to it, but it rings sexist to her. "You, as a woman," Ramona says, "are expected to do all of this work prior to being with the partner, and then you have to set your partner up for success." She would prefer if partners join the conversation, suggesting things they could do to help you feel comfortable, safe, and pleasurable. They could ask questions like, "Would you be open to doing this activity?" or "Would you like me to stimulate you in this way?" or "What if I change this?"

Ramona has seen many health professionals for her issues with pene-trative sex, and tells me, "I've never once had a professional say to me, 'oh, what is your boyfriend doing to try to support you in this?'" It is always exclusively focused on her actions, even when it's partnered sex. This doesn't make sense to Ramona, or to the many other survi-vors moving through the process of having sex with a partner, new or existing. We are accountable, in partnership, for our partners' safety and well-being when we decide to have sex with them.

Sexual assault is most prevalent among people in their late teens and early twenties (college-age is the highest risk time).[1] It's also the age when people start becoming sexually active (more than half by age eighteen).[2] Many survivors have posed the question: If I've expe-rienced sexual assault before I first became sexually active, does this "count" as losing my virginity? There is a legal argument to be made— that sex and sexual assault are not the same thing, so sexual assault has nothing to do with virginity. But really, it is up to each survivor to decide about their own experience.

Alisa, a survivor of CSA, doesn't remember a time before the trauma. "There really was no 'before,'" Alisa points out. Since there was no pre-trauma era, there "was no learning about sexuality or sex-ual health . . . about my own body and how my body feels and bodily autonomy beyond the context of my abuse." Alisa found that heal-ing from child sexual abuse meant acknowledging that "there wasn't anywhere to return to." She couldn't locate any "cultivated wisdom" or find the feeling of safety in her body that she might have been able to home in on. She didn't have any preexisting empowerment around her sexuality. "It's all about building a new path forward," Alisa tells me of her recovery process.

Alisa is not alone. Many survivors, especially of childhood sexual abuse, feel their assailants robbed them of their sexuality before they could claim it themselves. Like Alisa, survivors may find reclaiming our bodies proves a lifelong process. When somebody is assaulted before they ever had consensual sex, they may or may not consider that experience their "first time."

I once told a friend, "I think that my first kiss after the rape was the bravest thing I've ever done." Part of this courage was about trusting a man to touch me. A bigger part was about trusting myself to choose a partner who I believed wouldn't hurt me.

In the beginning, every time my first boyfriend post-rape touched me, even my arm or waist, I recoiled. I wasn't used to it being a positive experience yet. If he did something that triggered anxiety in me—like taking a while to respond to a text or running ten minutes late for a date—I immediately started on a downward spiral: *I don't want to feel anxious because of a man. This was a bad idea. I shouldn't do this.* If I was forward and flirtatious with him, I became terrified that he would go on to hurt me, and I would look back and feel like I had brought it on myself. In short, flirting and dating were a minefield because of my traumatic history.

Before dating David, I spent over a year celibate. My choice—less of an intentional decision than a series of avoidances—was reinforced by my parents, my friends, my community, my therapist, every book I read, TV shows, movies, and many survivors I spoke to. I felt I was reducing the risk of being raped again, putting off having to address triggers during sex or with another person, and ultimately giving myself time to heal. It's true; by avoiding sex completely, I minimized risk and put off having to deal with some kinds of human interaction. But I was also missing out; I was also sexually frustrated; I was also drowning in self-doubt over whether I would ever recover as a sexual being, no matter how many self-help books I searched through. I knew I had to test the waters.

I tried to maintain control by taking it very, very slowly with my new boyfriend. I remember calling a friend, worried about kissing him, and my friend reflected back that if he did want to kiss me, that would be a positive step, right? It didn't feel that simple at the time. Becoming accustomed to his body being near mine and *not* hurting me, even when vulnerable, while naked, while asleep, all contributed to the feeling that he was safe enough to sleep with. Looking back, I don't think going slowly actually mattered—we could have had sex months before or after. What mattered was that I paid attention to what I needed at the time, and stayed away from cultural tropes about when or how you're supposed to approach a new sexual relationship.

I've spoken to many survivors with similar experiences. Being sexually forward can feel painfully vulnerable or even cause shame, and being flirted with can feel threatening. Though in my own life, I interpreted these fears as a reason to hold off on sex for many months, other survivors have different experiences. It is also common to become more sexually active, with more partners, than before the assault. While this is not in and of itself harmful, sometimes survivors look back on their behavior and see how it might have been self-destructive, or at least not helpful. Soon after a man raped her, one survivor described how she said yes to almost anybody who asked to have sex with her because she wanted to feel in control of the experience. In her words: "If I gave verbal consent, it couldn't be another rape." Eventually she moved away from this pattern—though not entirely away from sex—and sought out experiences that felt good to her.

Danika was raised with the mantra, "Girls who get themselves in trouble deserve the consequences." She believed that sex would only lead to trouble, so she was afraid of it, and the potential consequences like pregnancy or STDs. She'd been told over and over that God didn't want you to have sex, and you would be punished if you tried. She went to Bible camp around age ten, and when she came home she took her brother into her bedroom and tried to convert him into even deeper Christianity—he was three years old. In her house, nobody talked about sex, but it loomed heavy and scary: you don't do it. Danika's childhood home didn't even have romance novels—those were looked at as trash. She intended to stay a virgin until marriage.

After Danika was raped during her first year at university, she went from believing in waiting for marriage to thinking "fuck it," and having sex with many people she knew. She self-medicated with alcohol to anesthetize the complex relationship she was developing with sex, drinking much more than she thought was healthy. She slept with her rapist's best friend and his brother, trying to hurt him emotionally.

In retrospect, Danika feels he didn't care that she had those hookups. She wanted to turn sex into something that had zero meaning. When the meaning was ripped away from her, she forced it to stay that way: "throwaway sex" is the term she used with me. She described it like this: "You took this. You can't have this now, but I'm going to give it to other people." She was trying to take back control of her body and her power by sleeping around. Many people pathologize sleeping around as a negative response, potentially destructive. Danika and many other survivors like her have found that changing their relationship to their own sexuality after assault can be part of a healing process, even if their sex life looks starkly different from what it did before an assault. Sometimes, our cultural rules around sex and dating stop working after assault. We have to write our own rules.

Mainstream society sees the rebound as shameful, or harmful, or at least not a serious positive influence. But many survivors see that first-time post-assault, especially if it's after an abusive relationship, very differently. Being ashamed of something that has a net positive impact doesn't make sense. After an abusive relationship, I waited a few weeks before going on a Hinge date. I wanted to get that "getting back out there" experience out of the way, but in reality, I felt more like I was facing a fear. I knew nothing about this guy, and he had a common name; I couldn't even Google whatever I was getting myself into. I crossed my fingers that he wouldn't cross any lines and all but ignored whether or not I liked him or he liked me. He was serving a role for me, and I imagine I was serving a similar role for him.

I invited him over one night shortly after our first date. He showed up on time, broad-shouldered and looking a little lost in my security camera app. I opened the door to let him in. He came across the way he had on our date: respectful and confident. But I realized, with this tall man standing in front of me in my living room, that I was a lot more scared than I expected to be just a few minutes before he'd entered my house. Later, I would more clearly recognize the fear I felt in my tensed body even as my brain skimmed over it. At the same time, I felt a visceral attraction to him. I leaned into his shoulder; he smelled good. He took off his shirt, then mine, and pleasure washed over my deep-set fear, sweeping it momentarily away.

Sex with this new guy proved distracting time and again, and while we weren't building a relationship, his confidence and commitment to my pleasure made each time we slept together feel almost joyful, celebratory, like I'd achieved some level of healing I hadn't expected to have to deal with again. I told him what would help (tell me a story if I become anxious; stop if I say stop, right away; I don't like pain) and he listened. Every time he listened, I got back some of my trust in the world, moment by moment resuscitating my faith in humanity—or at least humans I might choose to sleep with. In some ways, I had: Sleeping with somebody after an assault is a huge milestone, one that nearly every sexual assault survivor wrestles with. Maybe a rebound guy isn't the healthiest way to date in general, but after sexual assault, getting back out there at all is a step in the right direction that should be treated as such. And sleeping with somebody for the first time after later assaults can be just as difficult as that first time.

Some survivors even believe the narrative that having sex for the first time after the sexual assault can heal them, enabling them to move on as if nothing happened. The reality is much more complex, and it's not so cut and dried as a simple binary. Survivors most often fall somewhere in between—and often our behavior changes over time. It's important to move beyond the dialectic and see ourselves for ourselves.

Stacey was in an abusive relationship for years, and her next relationship had all the makings of a rebound in the mainstream sense: somebody with whom she was incompatible in both short-term and long-term ways. But unlike the common depiction of a rebound as a not-necessarily-healthy stepping stone toward an "actual" new relationship, Stacey's post-abuse partner proved healing—but not for a reason she feels others understand. In her words, "He did not meet any kind of criteria for anything other than being available." This worked perfectly, because she didn't need somebody emotionally available—she wasn't emotionally available herself. They met on a dating app, while Stacey was in the process of getting out of her abusive relationship. She made a plan to meet him in a public place, telling me, "I'm always the person who imagines all the different ways someone will murder me" during a date. She made sure a friend knew where she was going and headed out. The man surprised her. He didn't touch her or overly compliment her. But he exuded a positive energy Stacey felt to her core. He made her remember that sex and relationships don't have to feel negative or abusive. They can trigger your brain to generate positive emotions about yourself and the other person. Even without touching, the relationship progressed. "We just kept going out, and nothing happened. He was just very interested in me. I could feel the fact that he was physically attracted, but there was nothing more than a hug for weeks." Stacey's desire for safety in a relationship is shared by many survivors. Sometimes our first partner after an abusive relationship just needs to remind us that relationships can be a safe space for us to explore.

After weeks without physical contact, Stacey blurted out, "I don't understand what's going on." While the abusive relationship still affected her, Stacey still felt like herself underneath the trauma, and "[I'm] someone who asks questions." Her asking for clarity on their relationship gave him the permission he felt he needed to act on the physical desire he had for her. He hadn't wanted to make any presumption before that.

Stacey's rebound was affectionate, easily intimate, and intense. Stacey felt his attraction to her, and his physical affection. She didn't feel he played at her level intellectually, and he wanted a different life from what she envisioned for herself. But the physical attraction was magnetic.

Stacey absorbed his desire and appreciation for her and noticed his respectful approach to all their interactions. He prioritized making her comfortable. "The compliments were great," Stacey remembers. "I needed the ego boost. I'm not even going to pretend like that wasn't great." Validation and affirmation after abuse can be extra meaningful coming from a new partner.

Stacey wishes people were more accepting of the idea of a rebound. Stacey wanted to be with somebody, but wasn't fully available emotionally. She explains that the rebound "was part of my journey to get to a more holistic place where I could access different parts of myself." This necessary stepping stone was central to her early healing, but it's not commonly accepted as part of the healing journey. There is a strong belief that a survivor is supposed to show up to a post-assault relationship fully healed. If we're not completely ready and available, we're not supposed to engage with our sexuality at all. But Stacey knew better than to believe that message, having been educated in sexuality on an academic level. She knew it was okay to start where she was.

"It made me reevaluate how I had approached sex," Stacey says. Her prior relationship was abusive, and her rebound relationship reminded her that her ex's behavior wasn't okay. "When you're in a relationship with someone who is sexually abusive, your whole brain reprograms how you understand sex, its purpose and your interaction with it." Those false ideas were deeply engrained by the time Stacey got out. She needed the embodied experience of sleeping with somebody new to begin to shake them off.

But their incompatibility felt increasingly noticeable over time. While the positive aspects of the rebound relationship were significant, she knew it wouldn't work out long-term. She says, "I wasn't willing to sacrifice my whole person to be with somebody to have that attention and attraction and desire." She lost the safety net of being in that relationship because, ultimately, it didn't fulfill her as a whole person. Stacey recalls, "you could feel the wheels coming off." The positive emotional context they had built for themselves in which to have a sexual relationship was driven by hormones, Stacey thinks. When the chemicals faded, there wasn't much there.

On the Fourth of July, Stacey said, "I'm taking my independence back," and broke up with him—it was time. She remembers thinking, "I'm not in a place where this is going to work. And this is also not the kind of person that this is going to work with."

Two years after her trauma, Leanna reconnected with an old college friend. Right before the trauma, she broke up with her previous boyfriend and became single. Between the assault and her new relationship with her college friend, Leanna was not having sex of any kind. "I remember trying a few things," she says, "but as the PTSD came up I was like, this isn't happening. This is too stressful." But with her new partner (and future husband), things were different. Leanna was living in temporary housing in a hotel at the time they got together and remembers all the fun making out in cars and the crazy, passionate early stage of a relationship. They were starting to have sex, experimenting with different kinds of sex, figuring out what they liked to do together, especially because Leanna had little sexual experience at the time. She remembers being curious to discover more about her kinks, or if there's anything they should both try or experiment with. She had a beginner's mindset.

In this positive exploration, Leanna learned more about her triggers too. She found her partner had to be extremely careful with any kind of restraint, and while all BDSM is built on a foundation of clear communication and advance planning, in her case that planning had to include how she could get out of any restraints without his help. Sometimes, in the middle of sex in their early days of dating, Leanna would have a panic attack. In those moments, it was essential for her partner to stop and extricate himself from the physical situation as soon as possible. In those moments, she was seeing the face of her attacker, not her partner. She didn't have outside help, like a therapist, and that made things tougher.

Not all survivors' first sexual experience after trauma is with someone new. Many survivors have a significant other or spouse at the time they are assaulted. This presents a different set of challenges. Abstaining from sex might become more complicated if the relationship is exclusive and a partner begins to pressure the survivor to be sexually intimate again before they're ready. No matter what a survivor's relationship status is at the time of the assault, the majority will eventually face the hurdle of engaging in sex with another person again. Survivors approach this challenge in many ways and tell me about not just the pitfalls, but also the moments of clarity that lead to healing.

Danielle, a straight woman, was stalked and sexually assaulted by somebody in her community. The assaults brought up other bad experiences in Danielle's life, and she began to blame herself for what happened. Danielle, who grew up in the 1950s and felt her upbringing failed her, was lost as to how to deter the man harassing her from touching her. She wound up with PTSD. Her husband, to whom she'd been married for decades, supported her taking her assailant to court, and in confronting community leaders. But when it came to sex, they didn't talk much about the impact of trauma. She felt alienated from her body and lost interest in sex with her husband. Eventually, they stopped being intimate. Danielle tells me that while she's talked to many people about the trauma, including therapists and her part-ner, I am the first person she's spoken to openly about her intimacy issues. The lack of a conversation about how traumatic events and symptoms of trauma impact sex can translate into relationships like Danielle's: directionless and sexless.

Just after I began dating a man, Ben, I was sexually assaulted by somebody else. Ben seemed like somebody I could have a future with, and I even felt comfortable sharing my early trauma history with him soon after we met. He looked great on paper, so I tried to bottle up the recent assault and kept seeing him without good communication.

Eventually, we found ourselves in my bed, clothes coming off. My brain and body were not in sync, and nothing he did felt good. At that point in my life I was able to communicate when I wanted to say no (it might take a beat, but it happened), but this guy assumed that because I had been sexually assaulted, I must be someone who struggles to say no. In the moment, it was difficult for me to suss out exactly what was wrong. I had a freeze response that I couldn't escape. Ben may have been trying to be kind by letting me completely take the reins, but he didn't hear what I really needed: to be invited to talk more openly about the impact of trauma, to feel safe being vulnerable, to have someone else take charge. After toeing the line, we didn't go through with sleeping with each other. I learned from that failed hookup that somebody expressing their desire for me is actually one thing that makes me feel safe. If I feel overexposed, as if I like someone who doesn't like me back, then I feel too vulnerable. If I feel attraction or sexual desire is lacking, my body interprets it as a potential danger sign.

From my experience with Ben, I learned that every initial attempt to have sex post-trauma won't go well. We don't all get saviors flying in to rehab our sex lives the first try. It's an ongoing process, and sometimes the people we choose to sleep with after a sexual assault are not healthy for us—at all.

Soon after she was assaulted, Lyndsey reconnected with somebody she had met online prior to the assault. For the next year and a half, Lyndsey was in a relationship with him. He didn't respect boundaries and actively manipulated her. He constantly pressured her to have anal sex, and she felt like she had to fend off his advances. If she asserted a boundary of any kind around sex, he would say, "I just don't know if I'm attracted to you anymore . . . having a boundary means you're not worth me fucking." His words struck her core belief—that she had no real worth—over and over again. She felt, for a year, like something was off about the relationship, but so soon after the sexual assault, she didn't have the language for it.

As the months went by—and as Lyndsey did more and more therapy—something started clicking: She had to break up with him. The buildup to the breakup was painful. He told her that all their problems were her fault, and demanded she get counseling to fix their relationship. She felt awful, but didn't leave him.

One day, he was home with her dogs. She asked him to let them out of their kennel or take them outside. Even though he got home from work hours before her, he refused. He told her, "They're your dogs, not mine." She packed her stuff and left that night. Sometimes it is easier to stand up for somebody else than for yourself.

It wasn't that simple, though. After getting her own place a few days later, she questioned whether she'd made a big mistake. Was her ex the only person who would ever want her, given her trauma issues? Even though he wasn't good at navigating them, he had been with her since right after the trauma. Lyndsey's worry is very common among sexual assault survivors I've spoken to. It's difficult to leave a known partner for an unknown future, especially when that person is the first person we've dated or slept with since a sexual assault. Their reactions to our trauma is familiar, even if it's not healthy.

It took a year after Lyndsey left him to get to a stable place. To her, the post-trauma relationship felt like a second trauma. She had been vulnerable with this man after experiencing sexual assault, and felt he had taken advantage of her. Her post-assault anxiety led to a lot of self-doubt around whether she should have broken up with him earlier, and she felt like if she hadn't been assaulted and wasn't dealing with that trauma, she would have been able to have a quicker and cleaner break emotionally. The trauma, she thinks, looking back, was too fresh to be in touch with what she wanted out of a relationship or partner, and she wishes she had held off dating for longer.

For years, Lyndsey did not see or have sex with anyone. Looking back, she feels like she needed a more protective period to recover. She realized she didn't have much of a defined sexuality, and the idea of "reclaiming" it didn't resonate, since it wasn't there to begin with. She struggled with speaking up and began to understand she had acted more passively than she wanted to in the post-trauma relationship. In the past, if she wanted to use condoms with a partner but they said they didn't want to use them, she wouldn't say anything. Feeling less in touch with our bodies and sex lives is often part of the journey toward sexual recovery. It's helpful to accept that our first time post-assault may not feel as positive as we hoped, and to make space for us to inhabit our reactions to what is actually happening when we first reach out for another person. In the wake of her trauma and post-trauma relationship, Lyndsey learned to set boundaries and communicate with partners about what she didn't like, but she also went back to basics and figured out what she was actively interested in versus just okay with. She found her voice. If a partner suggested they not use condoms even after she expressed her boundary to use them, she would tell them, "if you're not going to use one, then we're not going to do this." If she wanted to linger during a certain arousing sexual act, she learned to express out loud her desire to keep going. If she wanted to have sex but not intercourse, she learned to accept her preference and express it. The trauma itself didn't teach her all of this, but recovering from the manipulative relationship she found herself in in its wake put the spotlight on points of weakness she wanted to fix moving forward.

Not long after an assault, before I'd had sex with anybody in the aftermath, I found myself in bed with a man I had met a few weeks earlier. I really liked him—and I really, really liked that he had proved so distracting from the turmoil of experiencing sexual assault again. It was the early days of what I thought would be a promising new relationship.

Andrew was respectful of physical and emotional boundaries, and I wasn't worried he would have a bad reaction to a panic attack if I had one. I unbuttoned his shirt, and his chest felt warm and safe beneath my palm. His hands wandered from my waist down around my hips and legs. When he kissed me, my mind went blissfully blank. There was only one problem: It was just too soon for me.

Though I was relieved that sleeping with him felt good emotionally, I felt overwhelmed by the physicality of it. More than once while we slept together that night, I nonverbally indicated I needed a pause because I felt a panic attack coming on. He was one of those partners who didn't need me to explain anything. He just smiled and lay still next to me while I cried and tried to breathe. Meanwhile, I was mentally kicking myself for disrupting what was otherwise pretty great sex. I was also confused about why I was panicking. He wasn't pushy, and anytime I said no or even hesitated, he changed course. I later realized I could feel my body fail to respond to sexual stimuli that normally turned me on. I felt numb but desperately wanted to feel. The disconnect between my body and what was happening was alarming to me, setting off red flags in my head that something was wrong with the situation, when really, I was only a few weeks out from a brutal sexual assault. That experience of my body not aligning with my mind was alarming to me, and reminded me of an aspect of the recent assault itself. I wasn't ready, but I appreciated that I had tried. I was proud of myself for being present with how I was actually feeling, for asking to stop and riding waves of anxiety I could've just buried.

A survivor's first sexual experience post-assault may be a positive or negative one or, most often, somewhere in between—an equal or more important sexual milestone compared to having sex for the first time, for many. Honoring the impact of that initial experience, both in significance and in how it affects us moving forward, helps us navigate the world of sex and relationships post-trauma. We can learn a lot from a first time, even if it doesn't resemble future sexual encounters. Staying present in our own bodies and lived experience helps us advocate for what we want, set future boundaries, and engage with sex moving forward. While sex after sexual assault isn't as simple as saying yes or no to someone (or any particular thing we do together), locating our voice in the presence of another person is a skill that translates into future sexual encounters for the rest of our lives. Luckily, we likely have many more opportunities to practice.

CHAPTER 7

Survivors on Consent

AFTER THE END of a taxing relationship, I met someone new on a dating app. Gabriel and I met for beers and took a walk on a summer night in Texas. On the way home I decided I wanted to see him again. Gabriel came over the next night, and after a quick tour we went upstairs and lay down in my bed.

Almost immediately, Gabriel struggled to navigate my trauma response to sex. Soon, I needed to press pause. I decided to share some of my trauma history as a way of framing my needs, but Gabriel balked, unsure how to respond. So, I tried to only share trauma-related information with him that felt relevant to us hooking up. After kissing for a while—warming back up—Gabriel got a little rougher than I was expecting. A wave of trauma-fueled anxiety began to hit me. I noticed, in the back of my mind, that I was starting to physically freeze in place. Before I'd fully seized up, and before I'd indicated anything was wrong out loud, Gabriel pulled out and said "Hey, let's stop." The panic attack that might have arrived never had a chance to start. I exhaled.

"What made you stop?" I asked.

"You seemed like you were in pain."

As he said it, I began to register pain from what we were just doing. "How did you notice that? I didn't even notice it yet."

Gabriel looked me in the eye and shrugged. "I could just tell," he said. I began to notice tension through my body. I unclenched my fist.

I'd never noticed somebody be so good at reading body language, and Gabriel didn't realize that what he'd done was unusual. I wasn't sure how to describe what happened. I, like many others, do not remember being explicitly taught about consent, or like Gabriel demonstrated, embodied consent. What I do remember learning was about the legal definition of it, a system of verbal yeses and nos designed to keep us safe. When I started having sex, I found this legal system confusing and not very useful. What happens when I need a moment to think? What happens when my physiological response to a trigger overwhelms my ability to speak? What happens when my partner notices something before I register it enough to say something? Then I talked to Stacey.

The consent educator from previous chapters, Stacey tells me about the difference between the legal definition of consent, which is about sexual violence and preventing crime, and the framework of consent that is useful in daily life, in relationships. She describes the difference as the "court level" and the "human level" of consent. To her, consent at a human level centers on empathy. When she learns about somebody else's desires or boundaries, she tries to consider how they would affect her if they were hers.

When Stacey was growing up, she remembers learning about consent only in passing. In school she learned it was a mandatory part of sex, but it didn't really mean anything to her. She says that overall, growing up she thought "consent is not cool." In the model of consent she absorbed as a young person, one person (usually a man) had sexual agency and the other didn't—they just said yes or no to the first person's demands. Consent was about gatekeeping. You were supposed to be able to safeguard your body, but not necessarily ask for what you wanted.

Later, Stacey's concept of consent was made complicated by experiencing a partner that used manipulative language in the context of abuse—by telling her that her boundaries were unreasonable. Stacey struggled to identify which were the boundaries she had that were hard lines versus more flexible areas. Going against her values was a no, but if her new partner left a wet towel on the ground again? She could accept that. Not every little thing was a huge violation.

Consent has become a buzz word since the #MeToo era. In the media and sex education, consent is typically presented in legal terms: "A freely given agreement to the conduct at issue by a competent person. An expression of lack of consent through words or conduct means there is no consent. Lack of verbal or physical resistance does not constitute consent."[1] The definition varies state to state, but often boils down to: Were they able to give consent, what did they say, and/ or did they physically resist? However, the public discussion of consent often zeroes in on a single question: Did they say no?

Some organizations, like Planned Parenthood, advocate for a positive definition of consent: freely given, reversible, informed, enthusiastic, and specific.[2] This definition focuses on helping people have conversations about consent and building a definition that functions and shifts within a sexual relationship. However, both the legal definition and this "functional" definition are focused on what potential victims of violence can do to prevent assault—basically, communication as violence prevention. What would consent look like if we moved past that baseline requirement for consent and refocused on how consent can be enacted between partners as a way of improving our sex lives? What if we focused on partners' responsibilities for checking in, not just our responsibilities to assert? What could consent and checking in look like outside of verbal communication?

While having a specific, enforceable legal definition of consent is essential for public safety and criminal conviction, the current conversation often fails to capture what actually happens behind closed doors. Rather than looking at consent from the question of what *not* to do, this chapter examines the positive definitions of consent that survivors have developed to ensure not only safety but also pleasure and play in their sex lives.

When thinking about what we do or don't want sexually—and therefore, what kind of consent we are comfortable giving—a lot of survivors feel pressured to fall into categories or stereotypes, hats to try on to help us figure out what we want. Many of us encounter the idea that we can be "prudes" (say no to sex post-assault) or "promiscuous" (say yes to sex post-assault). These stereotypes don't come from nowhere. In fact, both are rooted in real phenomena survivors may experience. One symptom of trauma can be avoidance of anything that reminds us of a traumatic event. Since sex crimes involve forced sex acts, it's not uncommon for survivors to try to avoid sex and their sexuality completely. But some survivors have more sex than they did before the assault. One survivor felt that if she actively pursued sex and said yes as often as possible, it would erase the time she said no and was ignored.

Sometimes, we play with the idea of sexual boundaries and consent. A man I slept with would act as if he was about to jump to the next level—spreading my legs or sliding a bra strap down—but always waited for an actual, verbal "yes" before taking that next step. The power play between us was one of my favorite parts of hooking up with him, but it was built on an understanding that he did actually need to ask out loud.

In a collared relationship with her current partner, Lexi went out in public with a collar on. A random man walked up to her, reached out, and grabbed her by the throat in a chokehold, wrapping his fingers around her neck. "You look like you'd like that," he said. Lexi was furious. Even if he really did think she would like that, he needed to ask first. Just because somebody likes a certain sex act or even a person doesn't mean anybody is exempt from consent communication.

Matthew described the lack of a cultural narrative around sexual abuse against men, especially queer men. In his experience, "the ideas of consent are a lot more murky for gay men, especially in environments that have a lot of drugs or alcohol." He found that these situations felt "blurry" to him, and he felt less comfortable saying "no." He felt pressure to be down for anything, which he associated with asserting his sexuality. For a long time after he was assaulted, he didn't want to say no because he believed his sexual partner would disregard what he said no matter what. He's not the only survivor with this attitude. There's a lot of fear of being assaulted again that goes hand in hand with figuring out consent in sexual relationships. Sometimes, saying yes to everything can feel like a way to avoid a partner having the chance to ignore a no. If we don't state our boundaries, though, we lose our chance to have a partner respect them—and be comfortable during an encounter.

Initially, Lyndsey didn't have good emotional regulation around expressing her boundaries, and might have an angry outburst. But over time, she was able to ask to slow down, to pause, and to explain why her boundaries were important and a big deal. Her desire for boundaries hasn't faded—if anything, her communication around boundaries has made her feel stronger. Before the assault, Lyndsey felt like if a man was sleeping with her, that defined her value to him, and she was too insecure to put up boundaries around the experience, because it felt like a blow to her self-esteem. Ultimately, after the trauma, Lyndsey felt confident enough to tell partners they could take it or leave it. She didn't need outside validation that her boundaries were worth upholding, or that her worth was defined by whether or not she slept with any particular person.

By the time she met her now husband, Lyndsey felt she was at her most confident, in her boundaries and her sexual identity. She knew she wanted him to be her life partner because he never tried to push her boundaries.

Lexi has noticed, while scrolling through men's profiles on dating apps with her partner, that many men put on their profile "Consent is important." She says, "First of all, it's actually mandatory. It's not important. It's required." The way those men are throwing around the term makes her question if they really know what consent even means. It's not just about people speaking up on their own behalf. Having consent also means that "you are showing up in a way that makes people feel safe enough to articulate actual consent to you, and to revoke consent from you." Consent isn't a value or an attitude that gives hooking up a sexy vibe; it's a guiding force that should serve as the container for every encounter. Plus, she recognizes that "it's not taught, and nobody ever hears about it." She thinks this is one reason turning to the kink community feels so safe for her. Kink is built around safety. It's everything she never got in sex ed.

Ignacio has been going to play parties for decades, and eventually started organizing them themself. Ignacio is proud in particular of organizing play parties that were multiracial and felt safe to all participants—of every age, every size. At one party, they witnessed a trans participant, who had recently been gay bashed by three guys, ask to work out that scene in the safe space of the party. They hoped, by playing out the scene in a way they could control, they could start to shift the narrative. That person got to choose everything: whether or not they would fight back, win, lose, act out a different role in the scene, lay down and take it, scream—anything. Watching that scene unfold, Ignacio, the viewer, cried. Even for an onlooker, it was intense.

Ignacio started to unpack their own abuse this way. They engaged in age play as a healing modality around childhood sexual abuse for over ten years. Doing this kind of work around their abuse was an exercise in specific, applied consent: They made every decision when it came to those created scenes. Ignacio was able to work through the abuse dozens of times, explaining that "Instead of trying to ignore it, I walked right into it." They had already been reexperiencing the abuse through nightmares and PTSD symptoms; why not try reexperiencing the event in a more controlled environment?

Every time Ignacio rewrote the script of the scene, they changed details of what happened: their gender, what they wore, what each person said, what the beginning, middle, and end consisted of. Having the ability to make those changes shifted how Ignacio viewed power and control in the rest of their life. Ignacio thinks sexual play can be a particularly helpful way for those who may not have had a traditional outlet to speak about abuse, process it: "This is the thing that happened, and this is how it hurt me." This openness helped Ignacio get emotionally unstuck. Perhaps most importantly, play like Ignacio experienced allows survivors to create a world where other people—acting as bystanders or abusers—will listen to you.

Ignacio, in general, has found kink to be healing, especially in helping them locate their feelings and boundaries, and later go back and debrief about what felt good, bad, and why. They don't know if their interest in kink is related to their experience of trauma, but what matters to Ignacio most is that kink ultimately helps them.

Alisa lit up while talking about BDSM and kink: "We owe so much to these communities . . . The sex that people are having in the BDSM community is so pathologized or shamed or seen as problematic, when it's the folks in these communities who literally invented our contemporary understandings of consent and boundaries." Regardless of what kind of sex you're having, Alisa believes a lot of our healthiest models of communication were developed in BDSM and kink communities, and trickled down into vanilla sex too.

Survivors of child sexual abuse might not have had a positive sexual experience before they were abused, and their entire sex life posttrauma isn't about regaining a past self, but rather starting from scratch. Alisa experienced sexual abuse as a child and didn't have a pre-assault definition of consent to reference. She found sleeping around allowed her to explore what she wanted and which forms of consent worked for her. "When I was dating around a lot and sleeping around a lot it was to really experiment around what does the yes feel like inside of my body? What does the no feel like inside of my body?" Sometimes testing out what a yes or no feels like with multiple different partners helps survivors figure out how consent feels for them as people, not just in a given relationship.

One night, Alisa met up with a man visiting from out of town. She'd had a string of less-than-ideal experiences related to disclosing trauma and asking for support from casual partners, but she decided to give a heads-up to this guy, just in case he reacted well. Without sharing the details of her trauma, she simply told him, "If I have to press pause, I'm just going to say 'pause.' Can we then pause and take a break?" She added that she was super into him, and really wanted to hook up.

This guy responded completely differently than she expected. He said, "Fuck yeah, of course. That would be a great time together." She realized that that statement was all the response she needed from a one-night stand. She went from feeling unsure about sleeping with him to feeling totally into the hookup, and closer to a "safe" feeling. Her casual partner asked what a pause looked like for her. She recalls telling him that for her, just knowing that withdrawing consent is fine with him helps her feel comfortable actually doing it, because she knows it won't kill the mood. Alisa points out "it's one thing to ask. But it's another thing to make sure people know it's okay to say 'no, no thank you.'" Consent isn't just about asking for what you want, but creating an environment where saying no feels like a positive step too.

Building on adrienne maree brown's conceptualization of "your yes makes way for your no," Alisa explained how to her, boundaries allow us to differentiate not just between yes and no, but between a "yes" and a "hell yes."[3] She says, "Boundaries actually allow us to be really into the things we're into, and feel safe so that we can be like 'fuck yeah, let's experiment or explore." She continues, "knowing that I have what I need, and you have what you need in order to feel totally into it . . ." makes her feel more safe and confident. Since then she's been guided by the question, "What would it take for me to be like hell yeah?" To her, consent isn't about identifying "no" boundaries, but making space to explore what feels not just good, but great. I found something similar, when I felt safe enough with a new partner to ask to try something new with them. When being vulnerable felt safe, because I knew they would respect my no if our exploration went too far.

Some survivors define consent in reaction to what happened during their assault. When Danika thinks about when she was sexually assaulted and how consent is supposed to work, she wonders if there would have been a different outcome if she had fought more, or differently. Was there some specific trick she could have employed to make him stop, to make him go away? She did say no, but could she have avoided the rape if she knew the magic word? Danika arrived at a simple answer: "You shouldn't have to do or say anything more than no," to enforce your boundaries. Words are enough.

Lexi feels that nobody explained consent in a meaningful way to her—it was more about checking a box, rather than the emotional ramifications of respecting consent, or not. Recently she appreciated the consent education given to participants on the Netflix show *Down With Love*, about the dating lives of people with Down syndrome. A somatics coach came on the show to talk to the participants about the ins and outs of consent, using the metaphor of choosing to share or not share a toy. Lexi remembers the expert saying: Of course you get to touch the people you love, but you always have to ask, and if they say no, that matters. If somebody touched your favorite toy that you don't like to share, how would you feel? If your partner felt like that about being touched, you wouldn't want them to feel bad in that way, right? Lexi believes that creative approaches to consent education and consent itself offer the most opportunities for consent to be effective.

Danika, fifty-seven-years old when I first spoke to her for this book, has noticed her definition of consent change over time, especially in the wake of the rape she experienced at twenty years old. In Danika's current, fifteen-year-long relationship, she feels she is past the need to use language to navigate every sexual interaction. "Consent means understanding what is being asked, understanding what is being offered, and actively accepting." It's not just saying it, it's understanding what's being said. Part of consent, too, is feeling "allowed to say that's enough." She operates under the rule that you can withdraw consent at any time. Counseling influenced Danika's definition of consent, which was very different in the early years after she was raped.

To Danika, consent always includes language, not just how bodies act and react. During one of our interviews, she defines consent as, "The person who says stop is always the person in control." The simplicity of her answer and the way it neatly rearranged very engrained power dynamics in heterosexual encounters stopped me in my tracks. Consent isn't just about a conversation, it's also about a full stop option always being there for whoever chooses it. Danika is describing the function of a safeword, a term drawn from kink and now mainstream, that can act like a talisman for survivors unsure what they need in the moment, but sure they need to pause or stop.

About six months after our first interview, I ask Danika about consent again. She agrees with her first definition, and expands on its impact on her. Reading stories in romance books, she has a visceral reaction to scenes that do not include what she considers full consent between the protagonists. She wants clarity in those scenes, not dubious consent, or dub-con, the term for romance books with those dynamics. Consent goes beyond the back and forth she experiences in sexual interactions; it's also present in conversations or media about anything sexual, for her.

Some survivors like to test boundaries and respect for consent before becoming intimate, to feel out how a partner responds. Danika describes her second date with her now husband. He was going to have to drive a long way home after their date, and Danika invited him to stay over in the second bedroom, or in her bed, but they were absolutely not having sex. "He did spend the night in my bed," she says, "and we did not have sex, and he was really great about it, really respectful." She points to that experience as a good test of her "no." He passed.

When Danika was single, in her forties, she always paid for her own drinks and dinner because it took away the ambiguity, the quid pro quo. She didn't want the expectation that if somebody spent fifty dollars on dinner for her, she would be expected to go back to his place and sleep with him. One of my friends who is a survivor spoke to me about her own vetting process: She cancels every first date and watches her date's reaction to rejection. If they respond well, she reschedules. If they act entitled, condescending, or rude, she blocks them.

Mia became tired of partners being cautious around her because of her trauma history. She wished they could shake their fear of a potential adverse reaction to sex. "I want to be intimate," she said, "and they're worried about what might happen, so we can't get there." She didn't want them to feel like they had to ask for spoken consent for every single little thing. Mia told partners that their hesitancy made her feel bad about herself. She felt if she was with a partner she'd been with before, and they had already done something she had told them she liked, it was less important that they ask a second time. It was then more important that they be responsive if she says no at any time. Embodied consent, where partners observe each other's body language and cues as part of a consent practice, would be more appropriate to what Mia wants: a partner who pays attention to her needs, but isn't all about verbal questioning. Embodied consent is powerful because when we learn to read our partner's body language and nonverbal cues, we learn more than just what triggers or hurts them and gives us the red light to stop. We also learn what turns them on, what works for us together, and what a green light looks like in somebody else's body.

Sometimes, sexual needs during a relationship change, and one straight female survivor, Laura, thinks explicit conversations about boundaries and expectations relating to sex long-term would help with consent in the day-to-day. At the beginning of her marriage, Laura and her husband had equal interest in sex, so talking it out wasn't a big deal. After having kids, when Laura's interest in sex waned, "being expected to put out became a problem." She felt because they were married and had certain sexual patterns established, they had an unspoken deal of sorts. Sex, to her husband, was one of her duties as a wife. She felt that something like a sexual prenup might have been helpful to establish at the beginning of the relationship, setting clear expectations that the sexual part of the relationship might change over time. She realizes that many people have the expectation that you have sex on demand in many relationships, but that presupposition is wrong for her. She thinks it would have been helpful if she had had these explicit conversations earlier in her relationship.

Because of her difficulties with sex after sexual assault during her marriage, Laura feels that talking to a therapist about sexuality should be a must, even in the early stages of healing, because outside of a therapist meeting, survivors are faced with the real world, including sexual pressures from partners, pressure to date or interact with people who are interested in us, and more. Laura wishes she had had more time on her own, exploring her sexuality, without pressure from her husband. She thinks she would have healed in a healthier way and gotten better at defining her own sexual boundaries and needs, which she could then enforce through consent protocols.

Matthew remembers that before his assault he felt like he lacked self-confidence. He wasn't sure why he was having the sex he was having. He believed that sex was an integral part of his coming out journey. "Up until that point," he says, "I felt pretty desperate to get whatever came my way."

After Matthew was sexually assaulted, he began to think more about his definition of consent. Now, Matthew views consent as important, not just for him, but for his partners, too. "If someone says no, I'm not going to chase them," he says. He was afraid of ever going through sexual assault again, but he was just as "afraid of hurting people as I was afraid of getting hurt myself." His assault led to a strong desire to make others feel comfortable. He notes that "it would be easy to take that experience and use it as justification to hurt other people," but for him, it did the opposite.

Ramona is very aware of how words can be misinterpreted and misunderstood, or even ignored. At a party one night, she invited her boyfriend to dance with her. "He took that to a much further extent than I had anticipated," Ramona says. He took her invitation to mean he could touch her *anywhere*, her ass, all over her body. She had meant they would dance face-to-face, hands on each other's backs, or end up kissing. She understood that type of dancing was his norm, and he thought he was doing what she asked. But she didn't like what he did with her words. He picked up on her body language and cues and apologized for making her feel uncomfortable.

Ramona has been sober her whole life. Both her parents struggled with addiction, which ultimately led to her father's death. She notices that partners act differently toward her if they're drinking. TV and movies tend to depict people going out on dates at a bar or restaurant where both parties are drinking, then they go home and have sex. Ramona has never had that experience.

Ramona's boyfriend got quite drunk one night at a party. He's usually horny when he's drunk, and Ramona enjoyed the extra attention from him, but toward the end of the night, she noticed he was really very out of it. Everyone had left, and it was four in the morning He was slurring his words but still insisting they hook up.

Ramona felt prepared for this moment. She told him, "As much as I would love to be intimate with you, are you okay right now? Can we check in and see how you're doing?" He stood up and said he was okay. They started to kiss, but she pressed pause. "I don't think that you can consent right now," Ramona said. Minutes later, her boyfriend fell asleep, but Ramona lay awake thinking. She had never been in that situation before, and she was not used to the flipped responsibility.

Consent happens in every moment, Ramona learned. It's not just about whether or not you're in a relationship, or what the usual power dynamic is. Everybody should be comfortable. Ramona firmly believes in treating other people the way she wants to be treated.

Ramona circles back to what this means for her own sobriety. Being sober means she's more aware of how she's feeling, which allows her to be mentally and physically present in a way she notices drinking partners aren't.

To Ramona, "consent isn't something that happens just in one moment, and then never happens again. It's always an ongoing thing." She sees consent as checking in and negotiating, even uncovering what it is that two or more people want to do. Sometimes, she points out, it takes time to figure out. But for her, at least, the more trust she has for someone, the better that experience is likely to be.

Many survivors struggle to communicate in words when something difficult comes up during sex. Leanna took martial arts classes years ago, and watched lots of professional fights. She noticed how, when the contestants were stuck in a painful position or wanted to get out of a joint lock, somebody in a fight would tap the floor as a signal they wanted out. "That's something we've learned to do," Leanna says of her and her partner's sex life today. That way, they don't even have to understand, let alone articulate, what exactly is wrong in order to ask them to stop or pause. She'll tap her husband on the shoulder or head to indicate "stop." She describes it as a physical language they have learned to speak together. It's partly driven by the fact that she doesn't always know what is okay or not okay until it's very not okay. She is learning to interpret the mixed signals her brain sends her.

One day, a friend who was familiar with Alisa's trauma history—Ignacio—asked her if she knew what her partner's boundaries were. Alisa describes her reaction: "It was like, crickets." She couldn't remember if she ever even asked him about his boundaries.

Just because a sexual assault survivor may have prominent needs, that doesn't mean those needs are more important than their partners'. Whomever you're sleeping with or in a relationship with, their needs must matter. Alisa reflects, "I was so used to seeing myself as the person who had all these needs, and my fear that my needs were so big that they took up all the oxygen in the room. There wasn't any space for [my partner's] needs, and that extended beyond sex, like emotional needs." Sometimes, being repeatedly told that we are the "needy" person in the relationship because of the trauma we have experienced means that we lose track of our partners' needs. Third parties, like friends, can inadvertently perpetuate this dynamic, putting survivors' partners on pedestals for handling our trauma well, even hinting that we are in a relationship with some sort of caregiver. This dynamic isn't empowering, though, and it's never actually true. As Alisa says, "We are in a partnership, and our needs look different, but they both matter and we both fulfill each other's needs—or do our best." The idea that we should be grateful to a person we're in a relationship with because they choose to put up with us is not healthy. Survivors have the potential to be great partners, and we should never be seen as charity cases.

Asking her partner what his needs and boundaries were opened up space for him to suggest ways to explore during sex that he hadn't previously felt comfortable sharing. "It made me feel like we were on much more equal footing," Alisa explains. "Everybody was in this together. Also it helped combat the pathologization that I felt like I was broken and fucked up. [Instead] it was like, 'no, my needs are different. But we all have needs, that's a human thing.'" Treating her partner the way she wanted him to treat her helped remedy some of the power imbalance that survivors may feel in relationships.

Alisa's friend Ignacio's advice extended beyond sex and into the relationship in general. Alisa asked her partner what his needs were, and realized that even if she was struggling the most with her own issues, she could still show up as a partner by offering him options to meet his social and emotional needs relating to intimacy, like calling a friend, or having his own space at home to be alone and center himself.

Alisa connected her conversations with her present-day husband back to the intersection of disclosure and consent: "It doesn't have to be disclosure of trauma. It can just be disclosure of, what is the green light for me? What is the safeword? What do you need after sex to feel good?" To Alisa, these are as important components of a healthy sex life as disclosing trauma history. Defining what consent looks like for each person is individual, based not only on trauma but any other part of your sexual backstory.

Ignacio, who has found healing and the building blocks for specific, effective consent at play parties, repeatedly uses the phrase "safe space" in describing their gatherings. I ask them to define it. Ignacio explains that they tried to create the safest possible experience at every step: how people hear about the event, how they apply to come, what resources they received in the lead up, how ground rules and safer sex materials got shared, how the definition and reasoning behind the safe space was shared, how safewords were talked about, and giving everyone in the space the platform to say why they're there and what they're looking for. Basically, safe spaces, to Ignacio, are created through very open communication at every level.

All of Ignacio's steps to create a safe space—a space in which consent can be exchanged freely and honestly—are translatable to sex between any number of people, whether a group or a couple. We can all create a safe space with our partners with as much intentionality as Ignacio, hosting a play party for many people. Conventional definitions of consent don't pay much attention to the space in which that consent is being given. But actually, that context is what allows people to feel comfortable enough for meaningful consent to take place.

CHAPTER 8

Triggers and Turn-Ons

A SURVIVOR ONCE whispered to me: "I don't know why—I was suffocated when I was assaulted—but now it really turns me on when my partner chokes me. I ask for it all the time." It's a question many of us ask: Aren't survivors supposed to hate everything about our assaults, especially when it comes to sex? When renegotiating sex post-assault, we have to ask ourselves what we want—and remain open to the answer. What feels good to our bodies and minds? What feels upsetting, or like a knee-jerk reaction to our trauma? And importantly: What happens when our answers to these questions are uncomfortably similar? For many survivors, there's no clear divide between sex acts that feel comfortable and mentally safe, and sex acts that remind us of an assault (triggers). Sometimes, during interviews, I told survivors outright to "tell me what you like"—because post-assault sex isn't only about dealing with the dark stuff. For most of us, it's a mix of triggers and turn-ons.

It's common for survivors to walk away from trauma with triggers. A trigger can be defined broadly as a distressing reminder of a traumatic event, including visual, physical, verbal, and situational reminders.[1] Ninety-four percent of sexual assault survivors experience symptoms of post-traumatic stress disorder two weeks after their assault. Nine months later, thirty percent still have symptoms.[2]

Sometimes I worry that disclosing my triggers could lead my partner to choices that make them feel uncomfortable, just to make me feel better. I don't want anybody to shave their facial hair as a precondition to hooking up with me. No matter how much I wish they didn't have it, I respect their bodily autonomy and try not to ask them to change their appearance to meet my needs. More often than not, I try to use it as practice to address those kinds of triggers head-on. I wait to have sex until my baseline anxiety over the situation is low enough to compensate for the things I can't change. But when those do affect me—an overgrown beard grazes against my chest and my whole body seizes up—I have to communicate about what happened. The other person wants to know what they did wrong, and I feel ashamed when my answer is simply that they look how they look. For a long time I prioritized overcoming triggers like these, specifically to avoid that shame. Now, though, I try to normalize it: it's okay to be turned off by reminders of some of the worst moments of your life. It's not a reflection of the current person in front of me.

To Lyndsey, triggers mean someone is pushing her buttons. Triggers can pop up the day after the assault or ten years after, coming and going. She says, "People think once it's been a certain amount of time, you won't have a reaction." But Lyndsey thinks it actually doesn't matter how much time has passed, and a reaction, like a panic attack, should be normalized even if years or decades have passed since the traumatic incident. It's important to normalize this for partners, too. Triggers are not a sign that a survivor is having a significant resurgence of PTSD symptoms. It might just be a blip, and that's normal for how trauma works. Lyndsey says, "Your healing journey is lifelong."

I have plenty of triggers that are sex-related; oral sex is a minefield for me, and kissing with too much tongue takes me out of the moment and leads to rising anxiety. These have been easier for me to explain to partners, because sex and sexual assault are often described as mirroring each other, in terms of physical actions. Sometimes, though, the relationship between sex acts used in violence and the sex survivors seek out later is complicated. Matthew says about sexual assault between men, "There's also not really a great cultural dialogue around the idea that the penetrating partner can be the one that is the victim of the assault—who can say, 'no, I really don't want this to happen,' and it happens anyway." He explains that in his experience, the assumption is always that "insertion is the violence." This baseline misunderstanding of what harm can look like confused him as he went back to the dating world. He wondered: Did certain physical acts put him at more or less risk for further violence? While the assumption isn't true, regardless of the gender of the perpetrator or victim, triggers built from specific physical acts can linger powerfully.

It's not just survivors whose triggers and histories can interfere during a sexual encounter. Every individual's past, especially trauma or pain, can impact how they act and respond even years later. Just like sexuality, our triggers—and our responses to them—are fluid and can change over time. That's why exploring sexual experiences on our own, without a sex partner, can help us better understand our own boundaries, and even grow as people. Communicating our shifting needs to partners and keeping communication lines open during any encounter or relationship is essential.

For survivors, dealing with triggers as they relate to our sex lives is especially tricky. Our bodies respond to triggers as if the trauma were happening all over again, bringing on hypervigilance, dissociation, flashbacks, and other responses.[3] It's a horrible, helpless feeling, especially if a survivor is already feeling vulnerable.

However, while some of us can't stand when our hair is pulled, or to be pushed up against a wall, or to feel a partner's hands around our neck, for others a sexual encounter that resembles a previous assault can actually be a *turn on*. But how could a reminder of our pain also create pleasure?

For some of us, it's important to talk about not only triggers and boundaries with our partners, but also how we might take pleasure from sex that resembles assault. It's not necessarily a bad thing, and we shouldn't be ashamed of something we glean pleasure from. During a panic attack, I mentioned to my casual partner that part of why I was shutting down was because he happened to look like the man who raped me when I was a teenager. They had similar hair and skin tone, similar proportions and facial hair. My partner took offense. "I wish you hadn't said that," he said, frustrated.

I reflected on the appearance of the men I had slept with. Most of them shared features with the rapist, especially their dark curly hair. I felt uncomfortable that I was attracted to anything remotely like him, but became curious as to why this might be. As I looked into it, I realized all men I had slept with shared another feature: they were either very tall, or very short. My rapist had been average height. Today I wonder if I feel safe being attracted to men who share features with my rapist with the caveat that since adults can't grow or shrink in height, I knew I would never accidentally sleep with the man who raped me.

The partner who told me he wished I hadn't said anything never saw me after that encounter, and for months I blamed myself; what I'd told him was inappropriate and probably made him feel bad. But ultimately I came to realize that I didn't want to be seeing somebody who couldn't handle the reality that any time I sleep with a man, I am reminded of the bodies of the men who've hurt me. I cut whichever emotional ties I still had with him and moved on.

For some survivors, the bewildering collision of pleasure and pain is an opportunity to explore the concepts of kink or fetish. While they sound taboo, kink and fetish are becoming more openly discussed and influential in mainstream sex. Even so, their definitions are fluid and dependent on context. A sexual activity can be defined as kink when it's practiced by a minority of people but is still generally regarded as sexual, like role-playing, spanking, or group sex. On the other hand, a fetish is an act that isn't generally considered sexual but is arousing to an individual, like foot play or specific attire. Communities have different standards, and so what's considered kinky in one space may be regarded as a fetish in another.[4]

For some survivors, figuring out what feels good and bad is complicated by other factors—for some of us, we don't like the same things all the time. There have been a couple of times Leanna tried something new and sexual, like BDSM-style restraints, and had a negative response. "Not for me," Leanna says, but she doesn't regret trying, even though it induced panic. She's happy to have tried out different toys and positions, including anal sex. Leanna enjoys the fun, "alternative" aspect and sensation of it. But it's much more likely to trigger a full-blown panic attack than traditional sex. "It can be uncomfortable or painful," Leanna says, "and you need so much trust and preparation going into it." At times, Leanna has said yes to anal and wished she hadn't, and they had to stop in the middle. Sometimes she turns down anal if her partner asks for it in the heat of the moment, but she isn't mentally there. She wants advance notice.

Leanna seems, to me, to be good at that connection between feeling like something's off and actually changing course with her partner. That back-and-forth navigation between her yeses and her nos took practice to learn. She thinks she developed that muscle mostly because she learned about herself sexually almost concurrently with when she experienced trauma, and she had to incorporate dealing with trauma into her sex life at the same time. Leanna remembers, "horrible massive panic attacks during the first six months of the relationship." For Leanna, like many survivors, the goal in the end was not to "abolish" panic attacks entirely, but to minimize their severity and make them occur less frequently. She is still exercising the muscles necessary to achieve that.

Leanna doesn't have many regrets, but she does wish she'd tried certain things sexually instead of the conservative upbringing she actually experienced. Her childhood makes her feel limited and inexperienced on top of the extra boundaries she's had to make because of her trauma. Plus, she's only been in one long-term sexual relationship after the assault.

Just as the definitions of fetish and kink rely on an individual or a specific community, survivors' desires vary and are deeply personal. Many survivors prioritize consent and communication, but that doesn't necessarily exclude a fetish or a kink. In fact, incorporating kink or fetish into our sex lives as survivors may positively reinforce our boundaries and priorities, and even help us to navigate triggers. Renegotiating sex post-assault can take many forms, and where we begin likely won't look anything like where we end up.

Gabby was raped by a man when she was a teenager. She avoided sex with men for several years after her assault. Many experts claim avoidance is a normal response to sexual trauma, and some say a period of celibacy, or a "sex vacation," can be a positive decision.[5] Of course, many survivors do not want to be celibate for the rest of their lives, and the vacation has to end. For Gabby, starting to have sex again after a period of celibacy was a rocky readjustment.

At first, Gabby said yes to any sexual invitation from men. She wanted "to be 100 percent in control of sexual experiences after the assault." Proactively offering verbal consent gave her that sense of control, because if she said yes, she felt she wouldn't have to deal with the trauma of saying no and being ignored.

Looking back, however, she doesn't consider these early sexual encounters, particularly those fueled by alcohol consumption, to be the fun, assertive ones she thought they were at the time. These encounters were her initial way of reliving and processing aspects of her trauma. If every time she said yes was really about rejecting the shadow of a past no, then she wasn't fully present during sex. Sex felt like throwing herself into the deep end of her pain and seeing if she could swim. Sometimes it worked, helping her to come to terms with her assault, but these experiences were never about building a positive sex life.

Alisa may relive her abuse, or see her abuser, when triggered. "I get really clear feelings in my body—extremely visceral," she explains. In her early twenties, Alisa tried to "power through" these intense triggered reactions, to block out what was happening inside her and continue having sex. This led to her dissociating out of her body during sex. Sometimes, she needed to fully pause when triggered, opting to stop sex and switch to full self-care mode. For her, that looked like calling on her support system and taking medication like Xanax. (Even knowing the prescription was there ready for her to take is sometimes enough to keep her calmer.) Alisa feels like triggers can become a "self-fulfilling prophecy" when she already has a specific fear going into a sexual encounter. If she's upset and afraid before sex, she goes into it tense and with a high baseline anxiety—not a state likely to lead to pleasure.

After going through a whole bunch of healing work, Alisa's old coping mechanisms—dissociation, powering through—stopped serving her. Even if she wanted to, she couldn't. Over the years, Alisa has tried to unlearn the shame and self-blame she feels when she dissociates during sex. "I think being in your body during sex is really powerful and important," Alisa says, but in the end she understands that bodies enact complex reactions to try to protect us and get through difficult moments in life. We can trust our bodies to know how to manage trauma responses, or at least we can be compassionate and understanding when our bodies respond in a way we wouldn't have chosen. In retrospect, Alisa understands her old survival skills, like dissociation, no longer serve her.

Later in her healing process, Alisa met her husband. While she had done a lot of healing work, she still hoped that meeting "the right person" for her, would cause the sex triggers to just stop completely, like in a fairy tale. She wondered if she had really just been with the wrong partners. Maybe her sex triggers had more to do with her choice in partner than anything internal.

For a while, she didn't have major triggered reactions to her future husband. Even though she only shared part of her trauma history with him, his reaction made her feel safe; he was everything she had been looking for. She assumed that she wouldn't ever get triggered with him. But, in her words, "that is a beautiful story that has nothing to do with reality." She distinctly remembers the first time she felt triggered during sex with this man. "I saw my abuser's face instead of [his] face," she recalls. The grief she felt about that overwhelmed her. "The reality that the trauma was always going to be with me, was always something I was going to have to navigate in my life, was a really devastating truth to come to terms with," she recalls. Not only did she realize on a practical level she had to deal with her triggers, but she also had to mourn the loss of that fantasy: that the right person could fix her issues.

Now, if she notices her mind wandering, or her body feeling off or "weird," her reaction tends to be less severe. In those milder but still difficult moments, Alisa takes a breather. She gets a glass of water and talks to her partner in a lighthearted, nonsexual way, making jokes and being silly to distract herself. When the triggers are not as strong, she wants to maintain a fun vibe while she overcomes them. She's still into the person she's sleeping with, still having fun, but maybe just doesn't want to be touched for a while.

Alisa's reactions to trauma are in flux. "It doesn't stay stagnant," she says, "it grows and it changes as my healing grows and changes. But accepting that there was no cure was, I think, the hardest part of the experience." Being with her husband also helped her feel like there was space for this kind of change and growth. Her husband has never made her trauma about him, only "like there was space for my feelings." This allowed her to feel less afraid of triggers coming up, because she knew his response to triggers would be compassionate, and that he would never impose shame or stigma on her the way other partners may have done.

If the conversation with a partner doesn't continue beyond the initial yes, triggers may still occur for the survivor. Everybody has boundaries when it comes to sex, and many survivors carry the burden of trauma-specific triggers, which can appear in the middle of sex and not just in the early moments when consent is verbalized.

Gabby felt this deeply, too. She couldn't stand a partner pushing her head down, or somebody coming at her from behind without warning. Pressure on her scalp, the unexpected presence of another body behind her own; she couldn't cope. These triggers made her panic, and in those moments when she couldn't repress her emotional and physical vulnerability, she often ended up curled up at the foot of the bed, unspeaking. Sex came to a complete halt. The onset of her panic attacks were made even worse because she couldn't explain why certain sexual acts bothered her so much. She was attracted to her partners, and she chose to be with them. Why, then, in those warm moments, was she so affected by the assault, which had such a different tenor? She didn't bother trying to explain her behavior to casual partners because she didn't think she would see them again. Besides, she didn't have the words to describe what she was going through, anyway.

Gabby needed to find a way to confront her past so she could increase her sense of safety in sexual relationships and experience pleasure in the bedroom. She also knew that dealing with her triggers would help her satisfy the needs and desires of her future partners. She didn't want to be prevented from exploring new sexual terrain with a lover because her triggers were in control. She decided to turn to a therapist for help through EMDR.

Soon, Gabby began dating someone new, who shared her sex-positive views. Together, they were able to communicate more openly about their sexual histories and desires. Gabby shared her trauma history with her new partner, and they agreed that during sex, whenever she was derailed by a trigger (less frequent after EMDR, but still possible), she would give him a signal and he would pause, respecting her cue. Before therapy, she had been out of touch with her need to pause. Now, she recognized it. Sometimes, in the aftermath of a trigger, she just needed space for her partner's caring, nonsexual affection. Developing this space brought the two of them even closer.

With time, Gabby felt comfortable enough to venture into new sexual terrain, beyond places deeply connected to her trauma. She believed that since communication enabled her to navigate the minefield of trauma triggers, it would similarly enhance her sex life beyond sexual healing. "If you can't talk about your assault or rape, it's harder to talk about sex in general," Gabby says. Difficult conversations that not only disclosed her trauma but also addressed her triggers and roadblocks prepared her for further sexual exploration.

Lexi believes that while communicating that you are triggered is an important step, providing your partner with tools to help you in those situations is that extra step further that can mean a lot in the moment. She emphasizes that this holds especially true if you are in a long-term relationship. Equip your partner with knowledge: What will it look like if you're triggered? Is there anything you'd like? A safeword can be helpful for prevention of triggers, or for stopping triggers from escalating. But it doesn't have to just be the survivor asking for help. A partner can introduce a protocol for what to do if the partner suspects the survivor is triggered or too overwhelmed to ask for help. Having protocols for a spectrum of situations can be soothing and create a sense of safety to survivors of sexual assault, Lexi says. The fact of being triggered—that feeling in your body—can create a lot of anguish for survivors, even setting aside the specific trigger, because it's the same feeling a survivor gets in the moment of the assault: nonconcordance.

For Lexi, being triggered feels similar to how when she was assaulted, she felt betrayed by her body, frozen like a deer in headlights. She wanted to run, but her body wouldn't; she believes she could have fought him off, but her body didn't move. In the moment of the assault, there was no script for what to do when she felt so trapped—nor, of course, would a script have been followed in an assault situation. But Lexi believes it's important for survivors to give ourselves and our partners scripts for when things go wrong during consensual encounters, so we don't have to feel that way again. If we make the scripts and protocols when we're not triggered—when we're grounded—we can lay a solid foundation for what needs to happen. The first time Lexi was triggered with her partner, absent their protocols, he would not have known to run a bath or take her to the couch and watch a Disney movie. But now he does know that aftercare, that caretaking protocol because they talked about it in advance. She has trained him to help bring her back into her body and her own sense of safety.

Scripts and protocols are just as key to generating hot sex as they are to preventing problems. Gabby's fantasies involved rough sex, psychological control play, and BDSM. After careful thought, she decided she wanted to explore them, so she asked her partner if he would be game to explore. At first he was resistant. After helping her work through her triggers, he worried that sexual experimentation would revive past problems. His reaction reflects a common belief: that survivors don't want to explore sex that has the potential to remind us of our trauma.

Nevertheless, some survivors like Gabby gravitate toward sexual experimentation over time. In particular, Gabby wanted to play control and physical power dynamics. Although none of Gabby's new fantasies aligned with her specific triggers, those broader themes had been part of her assault. Gabby isn't sure where her fantasies came from. In a different world, if she hadn't been assaulted, she may have still had the same fantasies. She decided that it didn't matter where they came from. So, using the communication skills they had developed around her triggers, Gabby and her partner talked about how to act out her fantasies. Gabby fantasized about coming home from work and that he would immediately start kissing her—slowly enough that she could press pause, but she was so turned on by this idea she didn't expect she would want to. Gabby explained the scene and asked him to take the lead more often. When her partner realized that was what she truly wanted, he got on board.

A decade after her assault, Gabby still navigates triggers during sex, but with practice, she's learned how to steer around them or pump the brakes if needed. She sees the combination of her strengthened voice and her partner's receptiveness to her desires as essential. Years into her trauma recovery, Gabby and her partner got engaged. They continue to explore each other openly and honestly.

Finding a supportive partner after sexual assault is complicated. Finding one with the same turn-ons might seem impossible. Some experts say that the real issue isn't two partners sharing identical fantasies and kinks but rather being willing to explore each other's sexual interests.[6] Similar to the way that a survivor's partner can learn to work with their triggers, they can also learn to consider their partner's turn-ons.

Sexual agency can mean many things for a trauma survivor. It might mean learning to navigate or avoid triggers during sex to prevent panic attacks. It might mean using therapy to overcome triggers so a survivor can relax and appear "normal" (i.e., unaffected by assault) in bed. That way, they don't need to dig into their past with every new partner—at least, not right away. Or it might mean empowering ourselves to act out our fantasies and ask for pleasure beyond what society says is okay to want. For some survivors, the very same acts that an outsider might assume would haunt or trigger us are in fact turn-ons. Embracing these desires—acting upon them—is key to sexual fulfillment and growth.

Alexis never could have imagined she would one day find herself slowly, gently wrapping her fingers around her sex partner's neck—let alone allowing her partner to do the same to her.

Growing up in a rural town in the Midwest, Alexis had internalized what she called "traditional" messages about sex, romantic relationships, and heteronormative gender roles. As Alexis describes it, where she grew up, "sex was not talked about in a healthy way—not in schools, and not in the culture there." She believed that a man's validation was the key to her worth. She imagined that she would sleep with one person—her high school sweetheart—then marry him and live happily ever after.

At first, life seemed headed in that direction. Alexis dated the same guy through her junior and senior years of high school and started college with him. Meanwhile, her sex life with her boyfriend operated under one rule. As she describes it, "Sex was about 'give it to your man,' to show him how much you love him." Their sex life was one-sided, and she didn't have much say in what they did together, but she thought that was for the best. For years, Alexis viewed sex as the means to secure a committed relationship rather than a mutually satisfying experience in itself. "It always felt like a requirement to have a sexual relationship with a person if I was attracted to them or wanted [a relationship] with them," Alexis says. She didn't see herself as having much sexual agency or room to explore. The "party culture" Alexis encountered as a college student, where sleeping with people was seen as "an accomplishment," reinforced her views on sex and male validation.

Partway through college, a man raped Alexis while she was drunk, in an unfamiliar environment, leaving her traumatized and confused. This crime was not part of her predestined story, and her belief in the balance of the world was shattered. Alexis sought professional help to work through the traumatic stress of the experience, along with a new friend circle who could support her. But she also experienced an unexpected shift. For her entire life, she had followed scripted notions of sexuality. Now that those had dissolved, her narrative needed to be reconstructed to incorporate the trauma she'd experienced. For Alexis, that meant sexual growth. In her pre-assault life, any sex-related experience that didn't fit her dream had made her feel ashamed, like she'd been the one to mess up. "A few days after the assault, I didn't feel shame," Alexis said. The assault exploded this old worldview, including how she viewed blame and responsibility.

The old rules she once lived by were so at odds with the reality of her assault that she needed to start from scratch. Alexis had casual partners and one-night stands in an attempt to redefine herself. Sex with strangers felt empowering at the time. They were brief encounters that she didn't have to "deal with" emotionally, she says. This was the opposite of the old relationship-centric narrative. Since she wasn't worrying about any sort of predestined path, she was free to explore. But Alexis reflects that going home with an unknown man after a night out drinking may have ended up leaving her with less control, emotionally and physically. Looking back, Alexis now views these free-wheeling escapades as risky, potentially destabilizing, even dangerous. What feels safe or not depends on the person, but any sex that risks endangering your health or life needs to be questioned.

It wasn't just her open-mindedness when it came to the number of people she slept with that defied her previous views. Alexis started to get into kink. There were lots of activities to try, but what turned her on the most was choking. Because it was something she had experienced at the hands of her rapist, her desire unsettled her. But in a consensual encounter, the sensations felt completely different. Hands around her neck had another effect: pleasant lightheadedness instead of panic, and then a rush of pleasure on release. Alexis said she was always gentle when she was the one with physical control over a partner. She checked in verbally, asking, "Do you like that?" Alexis enjoyed both choking her partner and being choked, what is coined a "switch" in BDSM terminology. When a partner's hands were around her neck, she enjoyed not just the progression from light touch to firm grip, but also the way it brought a sense of release.[7] Choking is sometimes considered a self-numbing tool because of the way it restricts physical sensation, but in this case it made Alexis feel empowered, inside the experience, present.

"It's like being an object—but you don't feel like an object," Alexis said. Objects can't consent, and consent was central to her approach to sex. She didn't play with choking unless "all those other boxes are checked," including consent, kindness, and checking in with both herself and her partner. Her check-ins were about not only safety and boundaries, but pleasure too. For Alexis, choking was a means to achieving embodiment during sex, or as author and activist Audre Lorde puts it: "The erotic is not a question only of what we do; it is a question of how acutely and fully we can feel in the doing."[8]

Choking is a growing trend in sex culture. As she got more into it, Alexis did some research, which turned out to be a smart, even lifesaving, choice. Choking during sex comes with significant risks—even death.[9,10] But some online research turned up best practices and safeguards, which helped lead Alexis to one of her central sexual practices: explicit, ongoing, open communication. When it comes to this kink, it's not an option to just play along spontaneously. Communication and a willingness to assert agency help sidestep any pitfalls.[11] Plus, being informed helps survivors better understand our bodies' potential responses and then decide if we want to try something, or if the sensations might be too close to an active trigger.

Alexis wasn't certain about why choking and being choked turned her on. Though she became more sexually active and experimental after the assault, she might have been interested in kink and choking even if she hadn't been assaulted. Many factors affected her sexual identity: her early education, her family upbringing, the sexual cultures of her hometown and college campus. Sexual assault survivors' sex lives are not solely reactions to assault, just as anybody's sex life is influenced by numerous factors.[12]

In fact, some experts think it's less important to identify why a sexual behavior feels good than to ask yourself if it allows you to be fully present. If the behavior is distancing you from your body or the moment, it may be a form of dissociation, or simply something you're not into. Being mindful of how something feels can offer more insight than an outside observer ever could. "Avoidance leads to a narrower life," trauma expert Judith Herman observes. Although Herman's work focuses primarily on the impact and treatment of trauma in everyday life, this message can be applied to sexual healing after trauma, too.

Alicia, the previously mentioned nonbinary and bisexual survivor, experienced rape at the hands of an authority figure in their life. When Alicia first reported their rape, they were silenced by police officers, who questioned their outfit and appearance instead of helping them. Alicia felt they couldn't trust anyone with their body for a long time. When they did have sexual encounters—especially with cis men— they felt unheard or expected to shoulder the emotional labor of dealing with their partners' inconsiderate reactions. It seemed like all they could hope for was better communication; pleasure wasn't even in the cards. Alicia described themselves as asexual for a while, and they avoided sex with others. They also abstained from masturbation.

Eventually, Alicia began feeling "strong attraction" again. They sought out partners with whom they could have open conversations and who wouldn't push them to engage in anything they weren't comfortable with. But at first, engaging in sex proved difficult because

Alicia felt ashamed. Even just desiring sex resembling their assault felt painful. Many survivors struggle with sex-related shame, and in Alicia's case, performing sexual acts reminiscent of their assault felt like inviting an assault to happen again.

In a culture that gaslights marginalized people and invalidates our experiences of assault, taking the word of perpetrators over victims, making us believe it wasn't "that bad," or "didn't count," it can be difficult to get to a place where we stand by our experiences and take our own word as sufficient—not just when it comes to boundaries, but what we're into, too. Alicia found their way to this place with therapy. They ultimately found that working out these issues also required patient, supportive partners who could help them work through their complex—and very human—desires and triggers. They noticed that many of these partners were into kink and fetish. After a while, Alicia wanted to engage in kinky sex, too, exploring elements of fetish, including BDSM practices.

BDSM isn't an uncommon choice for sexual assault survivors— *Vice* is even writing about its popularity. As sex therapist Vanessa Marin told *Vice*, the way consent is centered in kink offers survivors healthy coping mechanisms when navigating sex. Marin says that "Speaking in very broad brushstrokes, the kink community tends to heavily prioritize consent. There are discussions of boundaries, safewords, and contracts. Sometimes scenes are entirely planned out before two people even touch."[13] This kind of baseline control over the direction of a sexual encounter is appealing to survivors already struggling with trust and control, whether with their partners or themselves.

To feel safe exploring with partners, Alicia relied on some of the best practices of BDSM. In particular, they liked to use safewords, which can be used like traffic lights during an encounter—a word for "slow down," and another for "full stop," for example. These kinds of measures can help sex feel safer and minimize anxieties about navigating new territory.

Eventually, healthy exploration helped Alicia have pleasurable sex without shame or invalidation. As they learned: "I'm not devaluing my [assault] by getting pleasure from sex or getting pleasure from masturbation. My rape is still valid even if I'm getting pleasure from engaging in sex, in kink." Having experienced many negative reactions when Alicia told others about their assault, it took them years to accept both ideas as true: The assault and its impact were horrible and real, and their sexual preferences and turn-ons, including ones resembling the assault, were legitimate and nothing to be ashamed of.

Alicia's conclusion echoes activist adrienne maree brown's idea of "how we align our pleasures with our values."[14] If a sex act feels good and is in sync with our values—which may include things like embodied consent, kindness, communication, or playfulness—there's no need for shame or guilt about sex that resembles an assault. Orienting ourselves toward pleasure can never be harmful, so long as our internal compass accounts for those values too.

Sex that looks like assault may actually be much easier to manage than our nonsexual triggers, or even our partners' moods. For me, feeling suddenly in conflict with a partner, even just during a conversation, makes me intensely afraid they will hurt me. My body shuts down. My neck bends, my shoulders collapse, and my body tenses, ready for a fight. If a partner makes a joke, as a former partner did, about rape, even if it is not at a rape victim's expense, my brain freezes. And if I feel somebody becoming verbally controlling when inside my space—my car, my house, or even my personal bubble sitting in a bar or restaurant—I go on the offensive to try to minimize the perceived threat from escalating. These emotional triggers can be just as overpowering as those based on physical stimuli.

Alisa worked as a server at a restaurant that often played a song that was extremely triggering for her. She recognized that "There was nothing I could do about it. I couldn't walk off the job . . . I couldn't even take a break." She dissociated for the rest of the shift. But she was honest with herself: She knew she was checking out for a set number of hours, and when she got home, she would be intentional about reconnecting with her body. She held her dog, talked with a trusted friend, and practiced mindfulness. Sometimes triggers are outside our control, or things we can't "turn off," like that song at Alisa's workplace. These aren't triggers we can do much about, and being patient and intentional with how we respond can make a big difference.

Other survivors tell me about nonsexual triggers that get in the way of dating, like Matthew, who can't enjoy biking, including to and from dates, because he used to go on long bike rides with his assailant. Like many people, Mason finds if anything related to being gay or sexual abuse comes up during a family discussion, he starts to shame spiral. "It always bothered me that they'll never know fully who I am," Mason says. Lexi is strongly affected by the smell of her assailant's cologne, by the sound of footsteps behind her, and even the name of her attacker. Many survivors are affected by their "rapeversary" or the anniversary of when they were sexually assaulted—sometimes as specifically as a particular day, or sometimes a general season, or a week leading up to an assault. That time-bound trigger may raise a survivor's baseline anxiety so that old triggers rear their heads, or cause a flashback we otherwise might not experience. Survivors might not want to have sex at that time, or, as I did one year, might seek out sex as a distraction from the trauma anniversary. A location, like where the assault took place, can be triggering, and passing it by on the way to a date can throw a survivor off. When these circumstantial triggers show up for me, I try to treat myself gently, like I used to do in the throes of acute PTSD: being kind to myself, being slow to titrate into difficult behaviors or situations, and cutting myself some slack. I remind myself that it will all pass. All of these nonsexual triggers can affect sex, depending on when they come up and the resources available to handle them.

Lexi developed more obviously sexual triggers from her assault. When she was assaulted as a teenager, her assailant called her a slut and spoke to her degradingly. For a long time, engaging in dirty talk felt like "letting him win," so she completely avoided it. But one day Lexi realized that avoiding dirty talk was another way of actually letting him win. She reflects she wasn't doing something she enjoyed because of the assault and the attacker. Slowly, she started to explore dirty talk as part of her sex life with her partner at the time.

"There's so much healing potential in kink," Lexi explains, because you can recreate full scenes that were traumatic in a way that requires consent and is inherently not traumatizing (if done safely). You can change the ending, living out the scene in the way you wished it had ended (like Ignacio's age play), or stop at any time. Lexi says, "There's something very healing at a body level of getting to do that." She doesn't feel she gets this from talk therapy—her body needs to know she's safe, not just her mind. While Lexi finds BDSM experiences trigger her occasionally (just the way she can find non-BDSM experiences to be triggering), she likes how in BDSM there are ample fail-safes.

Lexi informs partners of her trauma history to help explain why she has a safeword and why it is important. She explains to partners that if she "goes nonverbal" and lies still with eyes glazed over, that's an indication that she might be dissociating away from a trigger. Her partner can then be aware, and they can navigate through the difficulty together, back to a place that feels good. They might ask, "Can we take a time out for a second? You look a little out of it; are you still with me? Do you want to do this? How are you feeling? What's coming up for you?" These questions help Lexi reengage in a way that doesn't ruin the moment, and offer a springboard for her to communicate her needs. Lexi makes the important caveat that safewords, embodied consent, and other safer sex practices are always contingent on finding a partner who is trustworthy. You can't build trust from only one side.

For sexual assault survivors, working through shame—whether in therapy or with a trusted third party—and finding the words to disclose not just trauma, but also desire, to a partner, is an ongoing process. As Gabby experienced with her fiancé, a partner can be kind, considerate, open, and supportive—and still not understand your interest in kink. Every survivor in this chapter had to work through this challenge with their partner(s) and realize through their own experiences that taking pleasure in sex that resembles assault is not, by definition, harmful.

In fact, kink and BDSM have a lot to teach survivors about consent and communication, which form the foundation for every interaction in the BDSM community.[15] It's not just about a verbal yes or no. Alicia described a practice they wished everyone would try: discussing the physical responses a partner can expect to see if they're turned on, like changes in their breathing, where their eyes go, or where their body bends and releases. It's the flip side of talking about what to look out for when somebody is triggered or dissociating. While verbal consent remains central, educating a partner about what to look and listen for when we're feeling good also attunes them to when we're *not* feeling good. As Alicia noted, "You don't have to get to a place where it feels bad and needs to stop . . . you can course correct." Attentiveness to a survivor who might be struggling with a trigger or dissociation reframes consent and turns it into a means of enhancing sexual experience. BDSM encounters also have the benefit of being carefully planned, so fewer distractions—or triggers—arise. A groove is learned—what feels good—and rules are set around finding that groove, which can feel safer to a survivor.

For Mason, too, basic vanilla sex is not a satisfying dynamic. There needs to be an additional layer. "It needs to be dirty in order to be fun," Mason explains. He doesn't pinpoint any specific kinks that are must-dos for him, but he feels like growing up in a conservative Christian household made a lot of things feel dirty, and he's grateful for opportunities to explore what that means for him sexually. He likes to adopt his partners' kinks or interests, and ultimately wants to have a shared "kinky, dirty experience."

Previous partners have not been as interested in kink as Mason. "They had a very limited idea of what sex is and should be, and can be, and I have a very wide [perception] of what it can and should and might be," Mason says. When talking to male friends, Mason notices they have a kind of "one lane sexuality" where they're just in it for simple, straightforward intercourse. But to Mason, sexuality is so much broader than that.

When Ramona was a child, she was "built like a truck—a very chunky young girl." She relished having physical dominance over boys she played with. She won every fake fight she started. As she grew up, that natural physical dominance disappeared, and she experienced sexual assaults that proved men could use physical dominance—or the threat of it—to violate her. BDSM has become her respite from the real world, allowing her access to the dynamic she misses about being a kid. For Ramona, BDSM allows her to play with gender dynamics and dominance—like adult playtime. She has played as a submissive before, but recognizes she doesn't actually want to do everything in the BDSM world that she has discovered through her research or come across in real life. Ramona prefers to arrange for men to run around her apartment, wearing a dress, cleaning. "It's the one time that I can feel like I'm not in danger," Ramona says. In other areas of her adult life, she feels that threat following her: on dates, walking on the street, and checking for footsteps behind her. She is careful about everything she does to avoid being assaulted: where she meets men, what they do, which friends she's given which information about the date so that they can follow up if a man abducts her. She lives in a state of carefully measured fear. The powerlessness she feels is in direct opposition with what she feels she gets from BDSM. She sees BDSM as a tool to gain back power.

Ramona has noticed the BDSM community is more flexible in its thinking about what good sex can be, because they understand people's limits and the difference between pleasurable boundary-pushing and what's over the line. Ramona thinks people who only have vanilla sex don't have the same exposure to these issues and ideas. That lack of exposure directly translates to a narrower definition of sex. Ramona sees sex as expansive, including whatever feels good, but also about intentional restraint to keep out what doesn't feel good.

Ramona compares the energy she gets from BDSM to the energy you might get from a live concert by your favorite musician. "You're feeding off the energy of other people," she explains. Even though in her BDSM scenes, she's in a room with one individual, there's the same electricity as in the concert hall. Ramona caveats that BDSM doesn't come with the same surprise or shock factor as she might experience at a live show because she signs a contract with her BDSM partner. Knowing what's coming is part of what keeps it safe. But she still feels a thrill, all through her body, that comes from doing the opposite of what society believes we should be doing sexually.

"People look at women's bodies as: we're the receivers, we have to take it, we have to absorb," Ramona explains. "As a woman, you need to be soft and caring, and you need to be a place for a man to land, and a support system for him," she says. But BDSM flies in the face of all of that. Men serve her. Ramona is particularly interested in exploring Black female, white male dynamics. She feels like her BDSM play is a way to subvert norms that are harmful—exactly how BDSM has arisen through history.

Since World War II, BDSM has been most closely associated with queer communities like Alicia and Ramona's.[16] Cultural anthropologists have also discovered that BDSM has deep roots, appearing in ancient Greek texts, medieval Japanese art, and other cultural records across the world.[17] Though BDSM is increasingly depicted in pop culture and mainstream media today, these depictions are often inaccurate due to lack of education in what BDSM really entails or consultation with subculture communities. While the internet has helped to connect members of sexual minority groups (especially for people living outside major cities), it proliferates misperceptions about core aspects of BDSM. For example, the popular *Fifty Shades of Grey* series overlooked how BDSM is built on conversation, consent, and trust—not spontaneous, uninformed, or one-sided encounters. Instead of relying on pop culture, survivors might be better off looking into kink communities online, or finding sex-positive resources.

One of my survivor friends, a queer cis woman based in the Midwest, used a fetish-focused dating website to locate safe, consent-centered sexual encounters in the wake of a sexual assault. On the internet, she could weed out individuals quickly, selecting partners based on common sexual interests, communication skills, and how they described their consent practices. She preferred this informed matchmaking to meeting strangers randomly in real life; it felt safer.

Many survivors find that disclosing our trauma history to a sexual partner and talking through triggers serves as an opportunity to learn about sexual patterns and preferences, about trauma or otherwise. We can explain to our partners how they'll know when to press pause, and when they should keep going. We can ask ourselves, "Why am I having this sexual encounter? Am I okay with the reason?" and with that data in mind, proceed.

But equally as important as recognizing a trigger is acknowledging how to address it. Lexi tackled triggers in a variety of ways. Her partner came over one day accidentally wearing the same cologne as her attacker. She started sobbing, her system flooded. Her partner apologized, but Lexi knew this wasn't something he had done wrong. She decided to work on herself beginning with the somatic work of titration. Slowly, she acclimated herself, building from a 0 to 10 on the distress scale. First she had her partner spray the cologne on himself an hour and a half before she came home, and then when she arrived, they would do something relaxing, like a massage, while he had the weaker smell of cologne on him. Lexi recognizes that that first step will look different for other people. For example, a massage doesn't feel grounding to everybody, so someone else might have to pick something different.

After getting triggered and going through the work of returning to baseline, Lexi thanks her partner for helping her come back to her body. She often explains what came up for her, too. If she wants to continue at all, she asks to cuddle for ten minutes then sees how she feels, which feels grounding. Or she watches a movie or curls up, or her partner draws her a bath. She learned this kind of good communication and protocols from her connection to the kink, poly, and nonmonogamy communities.

Lexi discovered that sometimes "dealing with" triggers turned into play. While dating her former partner, he arranged for her to meet up with another man. He was a primal dom, which meant he wanted to hunt her. At the bar where they met, he fell into his dominant persona. He asked a string of specific questions to set the scene and lay the groundwork for the dynamic. Everything sounded good to her. Then he asked if she enjoyed being slapped, or if that was off-limits. She responded lukewarmly, saying, "Sometimes," but then disclosed that it could be triggering to her.

He immediately responded that he wasn't interested in slapping, in that case. He said, "If I ask you for something and your immediate response isn't 'fuck yes,' we're not doing it today." His comment underscores the idea that early interactions require clear boundaries. "We're not doing anything that's not a 'fuck yeah' on the first night." If she wanted to push her boundary later, even explore it together, that was something they could talk about down the road. That validation of her boundary—and his adoption of her boundary as his own—made her feel extra safe. They ended up playing around with her running through a neighborhood, hiding behind bushes, while he chased her in his car.

Some people may not understand how this could feel sexual, but to each person, different scenarios are sexually charged. We often find situations that "aren't" sexual to be sexual because of outside influences (think: the eroticization of Catholic school uniforms, using handcuffs, getting chastised by an authority figure). If we're more in tune with ourselves, we may find other would-be nonsexual situations hot—in Lexi's case, being chased by a man in a car. At the end of the day, sex is really about play, or as I described it above, "adult playtime." Being in touch with what in particular we find erotic is a gateway to more pleasurable experiences. Lexi found it healing in light of her trauma around having to run away from a man in a car, because at any time she could flip the power dynamic and regain all control by using a safeword.

Taking stock of our sex lives—triggers, turn-ons, fetishes, and all—prepares us to experience pleasure and claim agency. We should keep in mind that our sex lives aren't static. Our sexual preferences change over time. Whether it's due to the distance from our trauma that time affords, or simply because human sexuality is fluid, identifying our sexual trip wires and pleasure practices is an ongoing, even lifelong, process.

CHAPTER 9

Pain, Pleasure, and (Sometimes) Orgasms

ONE AFTERNOON I found myself hunched on my kitchen floor, a stinging pain inside my vagina the day after having sex with someone for the second time. Right before I knew he was going to finish, I started to feel discomfort. In that moment, I knew what it meant—a couple of days of pain, exacerbated by a neurological condition I suffer from—but previous experiences have conditioned me to ignore pain if it benefits men. I wanted this new guy to feel good, too. I couldn't physically ignore the pain, but I didn't have to tell him about it. He left shortly after we finished. I didn't want to be alone, but the "rules of modern dating" often interfere with what I need as a trauma survivor. That happens a lot—all of the "shoulds" around relationships and sex we're supposed to care about, like being likeable or focusing our lives on finding a partner, go out the window when compared to the influence of trauma. Since most people I've dated or slept with aren't following the trauma survivor rules, though, I often try to appear normal, chill, like somebody who would be easier to be with than maybe I actually am.

The guy I was sleeping with knew about my trauma history, and I had asked him to check in with me if we slept together, telling him it made me feel safer. Whether or not a partner is understanding of how trauma affects me can mean the difference between a positive sex life and total incompatibility. Sometimes, it's harder for me to explain the link between pain that wasn't caused by violence and a trauma response. If something was an accident, why should it bother me?

Sitting on the cold kitchen floor, I kept glancing at my phone, hoping he would text me to ask how I was doing. I had been in an abusive relationship during which I was punished for being in pain and "inconveniencing" that partner, and I was still afraid to bring up pain, of the ghost reaction. I felt more comfortable sharing that I was in pain if explicitly asked. Being a woman, this conditioning ran even deeper: "toughing it out" and having our pain ignored is taught from early childhood. I knew this new guy didn't believe these things, but it's hard to overcome such deeply ingrained automatic beliefs. My phone vibrated on the ground next to me, and I felt a wave of relief wash over me. I picked up my phone, opened his text, and froze. He wasn't checking in on me; he was ending things.

In the days that followed, I was upset about the end to a potential relationship, the loss of somebody I had enjoyed being around. But I wasn't able to articulate the part that felt the worst, the most tender wound: how vulnerable I felt, in pain from sex with a person who failed to recognize my needs despite how clearly I communicated them. I was on the floor with nobody to help me up—literally.

Experiencing pain related to sex may feel familiar to sexual assault survivors. However pain manifests and regardless of whether it was caused directly by sexual activity, pain can be a trigger, cause isolation, and fracture otherwise positive relationships if communication breaks down. Sometimes, our bodies register pain from consensual sex as threatening, and we become afraid of our own bodies. Physical pain can cause a second wave of emotional pain that may become even more difficult to manage.

A survivor described that when she felt pain, no matter how slight, during sex, it made it intolerable. I've heard many survivors with similar stories: They became newly aware of pain during sex, or they began experiencing more pain than before their assaults. One survivor explained that experiencing intense physical pain during her assault meant pain during sex was a deal-breaker. Diagnosable disorders like vaginismus affect trauma survivors, but even accidental, one-off painful experiences can be triggering. Survivors tackle this issue from multiple perspectives in this chapter and offer actionable takeaways about dealing with pain during sex.

Ramona has experienced chronic pain throughout her life: headaches and migraines, digestive issues, recurring tendonitis in her arms. Between her own existing issues with pain and the idea she was indoctrinated with that women naturally feel pain if we choose to have sex (especially if it's for the first time, as Ramona discussed in a previous chapter), Ramona feels like a lot of her life "has been punctuated by physical pain" and it has made her less tolerant of pain in areas of her life where it is avoidable—like her sex life.

Ramona experienced arousal during an assault. Like many survivors who have experienced a disconnect between their mental and physical perceptions of assault (also called non-concordance), that arousal was deeply uncomfortable during and after the assault. To Ramona in particular, it was particularly disturbing because it was the first time she'd experienced sexual stimulation to her breasts in any context. Since then, she's had to recalibrate. Ramona has chosen to get comfortable with that type of stimulation and not link it back to assault automatically. Many survivors experience this anatomical or sex act–oriented link between an assault and sex, sometimes leading to a triggered reaction, or avoidance of that one particular aspect of sex.

Ramona has had issues with penetrative sex her whole life. She struggles to make it happen, and when she has been able to have penetrative sex, it ends up feeling somewhere between painful and uncomfortable. For a long time Ramona assumed the problem was her trauma history, but looking back now, she isn't sure she could pinpoint the reason.

It's been especially frustrating because she has reached out to medical professionals, therapists, and friends, searching for effective solutions, and was always left with the same, useless advice: light candles, use lube, and keep trying to relax. Ramona feels immense pressure to do everything experts suggest but it never seems to help. Sometimes, it looks like the professionals she's reached out to for help don't actually pinpoint the underlying problem, and are trying to mask symptoms. Ramona hasn't received conclusive answers or much relief from the medical community. But she did find women in online forums who struggled with penetrative sex. Connecting with people who shared her issues and frustrations, as well as fresh ideas for relief, proved to be a balm for her isolation.

Ramona feels very relaxed around her current boyfriend, but penetrative sex remains difficult for her. When she can't have penetrative sex, sometimes she feels like she's failed as a woman. But Ramona firmly believes that "if you can't have penetrative sex, it doesn't mean that you're broken." She thinks partners should be able to figure out their sex life no matter what an individual's limitations or boundaries are. "I need [a partner] who is down to figure out what's pleasurable for both people, and to dive into that and get really excited and experiment and have that be okay." She says, "There's so much to explore in the world of sexuality between two people than just intercourse." She and her partner have done a lot of exploration into what sex works best for them, and how to optimize for pleasure and minimize pain. "I actually feel kind of bad for people who think that sex is just PIV," Ramona says, "because there's so much fun shit out there to do [that's] maybe even better." Ramona has found many things she likes to do sexually that she can enjoy without the pain of intercourse. She makes an effort to stay present in her physical experience of sex, and to stay away from pain and move toward pleasure.

Ramona is keenly aware of the discourse around men's bodies being straightforward and women's being complicated. She believes this comes from men not trying to understand their female partners. Really, Ramona thinks that you figure out what works with every new partner. For example, her partner's past partners told him he is great at giving oral, but Ramona doesn't typically feel pleasure from oral, and she told him that. He was sensitive about her rejection, but she pointed out that her rejection didn't have much to do with him—Ramona says, "Each person's body is different, and it really is about the communication aspect, similar to understanding your own trauma response, and how that may affect how you want to be intimate." To her, knowing what works is so person-dependent that it's impossible to calculate generally.

Ramona feels trauma responses during sex, and it's layered with her shame over not being able to have penetrative sex. She says, "I would love to be able to just have sex like normal people," but then corrects herself, recognizing that there really is no such thing as normal. This has helped her recenter what does feel good to her.

Sex can be painful, and pain during sex will prove to be a trigger to many people. For me, pain related to sex, but not necessarily during it, can be just as much of a trigger. I experienced medical complications after getting my first IUD inserted that led to a lot of pain. When I went to the hospital, medical staff touched me without meaningful consent—the only way out of pain was to say yes to medical exams. I spent the night in the emergency room, thinking to myself the whole time: I was in this much pain because I'd decided to get birth control. The recovery from that medical experience affected my decisions about sex in the months that followed. I held back. I stopped exercising for months because I was afraid of triggering pain. Any touch from my partner felt threatening, because I didn't know where it would lead—not because he wasn't trustworthy, but because I didn't trust my own body. Today, going to the gynecologist or discussing health-care choices related to my sexual health proves triggering without exception. I am sensitive to where doctors' hands are during exams, even if I have consented to the exam in general. Stray touch is intolerable.

A lot of outside beliefs are tied to what we feel we "should" or "shouldn't" feel when having sex, physically or emotionally. There's a misconception that painful sex can't happen when you're in love. But at eighteen years old, Alisa was madly in love with her high school boyfriend. "He is really such a mensch, a sweet and wonderful man, and I was lucky to be loved by somebody so wonderful as my first real romantic experience in my life," she says. They were ready for sex—the first time for both of them—but couldn't actually make it work. "It was like a square peg in a round hole . . . it was so painful." So, Alisa went to multiple gynecologists, who unanimously suggested that she had an intact hymen causing the issue—but changed their tune when they realized her hymen was not actually intact. Everything looked "normal" to the doctors, Alisa said.

Finally, one of them believed that she could really be in pain and prescribed her a numbing cream to help reduce the pain. Alisa appreciated that she'd found a doctor who was willing to work with her and who wouldn't dismiss her pain or tell her to stop having sex. "But her response, or her solution, was for me to physically numb myself in order to try to have sex with my boyfriend. Talk about literally dissociating from your body," she says. Looking back Alisa questions why her doctor told an eighteen-year-old that she should prioritize sex with her boyfriend so highly that she needed a medical intervention—not to feel better, but to feel nothing. For years she believed that, since she saw her brain as broken, her body must be broken, too.

Now, Alisa can come up with numerous reasons why sex at that age didn't work. Since then, she's learned a lot about her body and about trauma. She's also had to unlearn what those experiences with those doctors taught her; an authority figure can create a second layer of damage. Alisa has worked on recentering pleasure, affirming that her pleasure should be as important or more important as her partner's.

After sexual assault, more than one therapist recommended I explore my sexuality through masturbation—as a test, before trying on my sexuality around a partner. The few mainstream books that referenced sexual healing post-assault similarly underscored the idea that masturbation is a key step toward sexual recovery and confidence if I ever wanted to seek out sex with another person. Basically, I was inundated with the idea that before I could sleep with somebody else, I had to sleep with myself.

I have early childhood memories of exploring my body, but at the time I was raped at eighteen, I did not regularly masturbate. Looking back, I think I was avoiding it because I associated the physical act with an aspect of sexual abuse I experienced as a young kid. My body didn't feel safe to me in general, and I didn't respond to sexual stimuli when I was alone as positively as when I got turned on when I was with somebody else. When my therapist suggested I read a book that highlighted masturbation as a key to sexual healing, I nodded along. But I didn't start masturbating regularly until years later, after I'd broken up with a longtime boyfriend. I got the first vibrator that actually worked for me—there are so many! keep looking!—and spent some time exploring on my own.

At that point, thrust back into the world of being single, dating, and figuring out how to trust new people, masturbation felt like a safe escape from potential trauma symptoms that would come up with new people. When I was alone, I was in control, and I felt less pressure to go out and date or sleep with anybody else if I could satisfy myself sexually.

Even when I started having casual sex regularly, or later got into relationships, I have kept up masturbating. It helps me feel in control of my sex drive, helps me relax and refocus when I'm stressed, and is a reliable source of pleasure.

Over the years, I've noticed a pattern: my relationship with masturbation has developed independently from my relationship with sex with partners. The two are separate, not sequential. I hope other trauma survivors can avoid the pressure I felt to explore masturbation as a prerequisite to sex with somebody else. Pleasure alone for its own sake is worth pursuing and doesn't have to be tied to whether we're ready for sex with a partner. And if you do have a partner, that doesn't mean you have to abandon pursuing sex solo, whether that's through masturbating, watching porn, or whatever feels safe and satisfying to you. By honoring your relationship with your own body, you're actually setting yourself up to have a better relationship with a partner—who hopefully has a strong relationship with their body, too.

By exploring alone, some survivors have restructured their approach to sexual pleasure. They focus on sustaining and increasing pleasure, rather than reaching orgasm. It's not that people *shouldn't* orgasm during sex, it's just that it doesn't have to be the end goal. (And sometimes, making sex about a goal at all can feel upsetting.) They often carry this philosophy forward into sexual relationships with other people. On the other hand, some survivors told me that centering a sexual experience around orgasm is empowering for them and communicates a clear message: My satisfaction comes first.

Survivors sometimes find that taking a step toward pleasure alone makes moving forward with a partner a more comfortable—and satisfying—experience. Others feel that solo sexual pleasure and orgasm is worthwhile for its own sake. I ask Lyndsey about masturbation and pleasure. She says she didn't feel shame while masturbating because she knew that alone, she was safe, and wouldn't end up looking back on what she was doing with any kind of regret or shame tied to another person. She could decide what to think about, what she would do or use to turn herself on. She didn't have to think about anything that might make her feel bad, like a partner's desires or actions. It's more control than she feels she could ever have with a partner, even an understanding one, because no matter how healthy your relationship or sex life is, you're never completely in control—it's a two-way street and requires mutual consent. Even trying to set up a sexual encounter based primarily on your needs and boundaries doesn't guarantee the encounter will stay that way. A survivor's preferred sexual position may work for their partner, until the partner asks to switch things up. Choosing to masturbate solo avoids any difficulties that might come up with a partner.

But eventually, many survivors will seek out touch from another person. Stacey's first partner post-assault, the rebound mentioned earlier, was not an emotionally close relationship, but it was a positive physical one, and recalibrated her body to the idea that sex could be positive. When they met, Stacey could feel her date's attraction to her, but he didn't cross any boundaries or even touch her. Being sexually desired without being touched more than she was ready for made her feel open to connecting to pleasure. Sometimes a prerequisite for feeling safe in a sexual interaction is a partner openly expressing desire for us in a way that doesn't interfere with navigating our trauma. Stacey's casual partner was very attentive, checking in with her frequently throughout hookups, and for that stage of healing, she says, "I couldn't have asked for anything more." That pleasure-centered physical relationship shifted how she saw her own body. She chose not to shut herself off from pleasure and reoriented away from fear and shame toward feeling good. After being in a long-term abusive relationship, her hookup helped her realize her sex life could be completely different.

A couple of years after we first spoke, Mia and I talked again. She had been single since her most recent assault, had never been in a committed relationship before, and still felt alienated by touch. She just couldn't get there, and even nonsexual physical touch from her mother could set her off. With women-identifying partners, it was easier. Since her assault, she hadn't felt as intimately close with men (the gender identity of her attacker) as she did with women. She found it more difficult to access pleasure around men than women. During later interviews, Mia spoke to me about regaining trust in men so that their touch felt positive, and she felt able to experience pleasure with them, but it was a multiyear process.

Alisa realized she was still operating under an old, ingrained habit: she was dissociating in order to keep going for her partner. She prioritized her partner's pleasure over her own presence during their encounters. As a heterosexual woman, she "had been conditioned to prioritize a man's pleasure" over her own experience. She wanted her partners to enjoy themselves, but at the same time questioned why she was sleeping with men who didn't care about her pleasure as much as she cared about theirs.

Mason finds it difficult to receive pleasure if his partner isn't experiencing pleasure at the same time. What excites him the most, he says, is taking care of the other person. Mason has a hard time receiving pleasure or being the focus of a sexual encounter. He explains, "I'm not great at receiving a blowjob, but I love going down on a woman so much, or a guy, too. It's my favorite thing in the world to do." This dynamic mirrors his trauma history, and some people have seen his imbalanced focus on his partner as problematic. However, he gets genuine joy and pleasure from these interactions. A partner once explained to him that being this way actually denies his partner the opportunity to be giving, which she wanted. Mason is working on balancing both sides of pleasure, and feeling the discomfort that comes up around receiving pleasure.

But sometimes it can take years to figure out what you'd like to receive—or what pleasure even looks like for you. Danika's sex life during her first marriage was only about getting pregnant. Her first husband never made her laugh. But as it turned out, Danika's love language is laughter: "If I'm laughing during sex, that is a good thing." Now, decades later she says, sex isn't about getting pregnant: "It's 100 percent about pleasure."

Stacey explains that when it comes to orgasms, she sees a pleasure gap: people with certain anatomy, mainly cis men, are always entitled to an orgasm. For other people, pleasure is barely a commonly expected consideration. Stacey knows from personal and professional experience in consent education that pleasure can become complicated by sexual assault. Ultimately, she supports the idea that we can all focus on our partner's pleasure to counteract the existing paradigm about which people get to receive pleasure during sexual encounters.

Stacey tells me that while the average sexual encounter is between two and eight minutes, someone with a vagina takes on average fourteen minutes to climax.[1] For women and AFAB people, she says, "your pleasure never mattered in the first place," so while advocating for pleasure may be part of the healing process, it doesn't necessarily have any pre-assault roots to grow from. Centering your own pleasure may feel radical, because it is.

On the other hand, decentering your orgasm can appear, or feel, radical. "For a long time," Matthew recalls, "I would just not finish in sex. I'd be like, nope, this is taking too long. You're done, so I'm done." He noticed that many people found this to be a turnoff. Partners took it personally if Matthew wanted to stop an encounter before he finished. He worried he was just not into the people he slept with— plus, he felt alone because he didn't know anybody else struggling to ejaculate. Matthew felt isolated even during his casual hookups. Matthew felt that if he wasn't enjoying sex as much as he thought he was supposed to, he would focus exclusively on the other person's pleasure. "That's definitely wrong," Matthew says of his past perspective, continuing, "I did not make space for myself, and I didn't feel like I had the right to." Matthew felt the chokehold of society's expectations: that sex should end in orgasm, or else it was bad, an attitude confirmed over and over again by the culture he consumed.

One survivor felt a lot of pressure to orgasm with her first partner after her assault. Orgasm required a level of surrender and release that she wasn't ready for in front of another person. There is an inherent vulnerability to orgasming that can feel particularly scary to survivors. We might feel shame if we don't "succeed" at orgasming, and shame is the last thing we should have to feel.

Ramona believes in shifting the goalpost from orgasms to pleasure. She points out that some people can't easily orgasm, so assuming they can is invalidating. Sex positive spaces, Ramona says, make the assumption that everybody's goal is to orgasm, and many people describe orgasm as the ultimate human experience. Supposedly everybody wants to orgasm, Ramona tells me, but "it's just not fucking true." In her first serious relationship, Ramona and her partner played in ways that felt pleasurable, but she didn't want to focus on orgasm at the time, and she didn't reach for that. Intimacy, whether pleasure-focused or orgasm-oriented, requires vulnerability. Orgasm may require a level of surrender and release that a survivor may not be ready for. It can leave you feeling exposed, which may be particularly scary for survivors. Ramona sees a lot of the pressure to orgasm as being mostly about proving a point, or performing pleasure. The journey-not-the-destination, pleasure-focused sex she prefers is about actually feeling pleasure, not performing it.

If Ramona is taking a long time to come, and wants to opt out—it's not gonna happen that night—she offers her partner a way out. To her, the goal is usually "to enjoy each other's bodies. The goal is to be present, the goal is whatever you want from that experience." Sometimes her goal is something she associates with intimacy and sensuality: being face-to-face with someone, their cheeks almost touching, absorbing them in all their up close detail. Looking into their eyes makes her feel connected. "That can be a very sexually charged thing," Ramona says, and "It can be a very intimate, cozy thing. It can have a lot of different meanings." Ramona believes there's a lot more she can access through her sexuality beyond sex itself.

Today, Ramona does want to try more of the sexual things she once wrote off. She feels her sexuality ebbing and flowing, and follows those changes as they come. Ramona was on vacation with her partner shortly before we spoke, feeling extra relaxed. When she removed the time pressure to come quickly, felt during her normal life, Ramona lost some of her nervousness. Orgasm wasn't necessarily the goal in the moment, but it felt like a natural time to reach for it, when they were both genuinely excited and relaxed. For the first time in their relationship, she came.

Leanna feels she had to go out of her way to learn things that other people's bodies learn "naturally" around puberty, like sexual exploration and orgasm. She felt behind, unable to consistently orgasm, and never with a partner. Before her husband but after the trauma, Leanna made attempts to be intimate with a couple of different men. She still hadn't experienced an orgasm, and with those men she would feel "a buildup of something" that felt good, but at the same time, terrifying. She interpreted it as something happening that she couldn't control or understand. She would stop immediately and cut off the sexual interaction there. It wasn't until her husband, her current partner, that she relaxed into the relationship and into the sex for the first time. Leanna hadn't had an orgasm when she met her husband. "My body just didn't do that at that point." She felt like he was a safe person to experience orgasm with, so they experimented, figuring out what felt good to her. With her husband, she says, "Not only was I able to experience an orgasm, but they got more and more intense over time, the longer I was with my partner."

Leanna has learned a lot since then. She's found that for about sixty seconds after she orgasms, she feels super sensitive. Her partner might try to stimulate her clit again, or try oral again. But after that window for a second orgasm, her body shuts down and goes "kind of numb." If Leanna ever finds herself building up to a second orgasm during vaginal or anal sex, she experiences what she used to experience whenever she tried for an orgasm: her body recognizes something unfamiliar, and reacts with caution. It's a mental and physical block for Leanna. She has to slow things down. "I would love to just be having multiple orgasms all over the place," Leanna says, "but for now it just seems like my body is like, you know what? One is good for now. We're happy." The second orgasm, something our culture lusts after, highlights that feeling of not being safe for her, and exacerbates anxieties. Instead of pressuring herself to achieve that second orgasm, she backs off of it and into safety. Many survivors search for that sense of safety beyond anything else—if sex feels safe, it was good, regardless of whether it was satisfying. Sometimes satisfying is out of reach, like if our fight or flight is too high or we're sleeping with a new person. We get to set our own goals, and if our main or sole goal is safety, that is just as worthwhile as having an orgasm.

Survivors are empowered to access what we want out of sex, and to maneuver our way out of sensations we don't want to feel, like pain. Neither requires a partner. If you are alone you can masturbate to experience sexual pleasure, like Lyndsey. If you are alone and in pain, you can reach out to support for managing that pain, like Ramona. And if you are in a relationship, pain, pleasure, and potential orgasm can be seen as opportunities to connect. Just as we are responsible for advocating for our own pleasure and orgasm, we are empowered to manage pain that comes up from sex—but we don't have to do it alone. Asking for help from partners, professionals, or loved ones is a skill we can cultivate that paves the way for future pleasure. On the other hand, learning to manage difficulties that come up from sex on our own is a valuable tool that will help us better live out our own sexual agency and be better partners too. It's a skill that can help us manage other issues that come up related to sex and sexual assault, from mental illness to STI status to pregnancy.

CHAPTER 10

Overcoming Setbacks

AFTER I WAS raped as a teenager, my doctor put me on a medication to help me sleep at night. It was meant to help me through PTSD treatment, but no doctor took me off of the medication—for years. Four years after first swallowing one of those pills, I decided to come off of it alone. The withdrawal symptoms, which lasted over a month, strained my long-term relationship immensely, interrupting not just our daily life but both of our careers and plans for that season. While my partner, David, was supportive, I began to doubt, in my post-medicated state, if he was the right partner for me for the long term. Everything seemed to be happening at once: the withdrawal symptoms, the life season transition from student to adult, the dulled, medicated state to somebody who was fully awake to her own life. It dawned on me that the relationship I was in, loving as it was, would not last.

I had never broken up with anybody, and I put it off for months because I was afraid I'd never find anybody as good at "dealing with" my trauma as him. David was understanding, patient, and good at listening. He rarely pushed a boundary in the five years we were together, and if he did want something different from me, it was always asked as a kindly phrased question. But in other areas of our life together, we were not in alignment. Where we wanted to live, what I wanted to

187

do with my time and career, what we wanted out of life in many major ways, were completely out of sync. We'd given it our best shot, and at the end of the day, he was comfortable and I was unhappy. I knew it was up to me to break up with him or I would stay stuck living inside somebody else's life forever. But every time I had a conversation with him about the future, the idea of having to navigate dating and sex with my trauma history seemed an insurmountable barrier. I had no idea how to do it; I'd only slept with David after I was raped. And I knew from trial and error with friends that not everybody handles conversations about trauma well, let alone trauma and sex.

Many survivors express a specific fear: They do not want to end a relationship with somebody who has been particularly adept at navigating their trauma. They believed that they would never find anybody better at that. Even if a relationship wasn't working for other reasons, they are hesitant to break up with someone or particularly devastated if that person breaks up with them. I stayed in the relationship with David an entire year after realizing I wanted to leave because I was worried I wouldn't find somebody else who could "handle" my trauma.

I reached a breaking point and ended things with him, launching myself into the rest of my life. What I found surprised me: other partners proved not just up to David's standard, but actually better at dealing with trauma. I learned I didn't just want a partner who could navigate my trauma as David had; I wanted a partner who knew how to openly express desire for me in a way that didn't interfere with navigating trauma. I wanted pleasure and play, not just someone who could help me wade through pain. There are so many ways for a partner to work with a partner's trauma. As I've gotten older, I found that many partners my age had already navigated sex with a trauma survivor, and had some baseline understanding of what I needed. But it wasn't just older partners who I found the most success with. I dated one partner, five years younger than me, for a year. He was so good at navigating sex post-assault that when he broke up with me, I found myself mourning not just the end of the relationship, but the loss of someone that skilled at handling trauma. But I remembered how afraid I'd been at the end of my first serious relationship and was reassured that I could find somebody just as skillful as the man who'd just dumped me. I became focused on finding a solid partner who could meet my needs around trauma navigation and stability. I could move forward, to somebody new.

No matter how much effort we put into healing, no matter how far we've come, survivors still encounter roadblocks in our sex lives, simply because we're human. Medical issues, social issues, sexual issues: for many survivors, these are felt through the lens of sexual trauma. We may get rejected or dumped, lied to or cheated on—or we cheat, lie, or break up with somebody ourselves. These are common experiences for anyone pursuing sexual relationships, but having a traumatic history may intensify these typical human experiences. Then right when we think we've reached a place of healing, we get hurt again—sometimes, raped again.

Many of us seek to reach a state where we are "healed." That can mean something different to each of us but always implies the same thing: There will come a time when the healing is done and we won't be affected by trauma anymore. But Lexi tells me that she thinks talking about being "healed" in the past tense is dangerous. Then, if we do get triggered, we might feel like we're having a kind of relapse. Lexi says, "The expectation that there's going to be a day where it just never bothers you again feels problematic." We can do all the work, but trauma lives inside us, and no matter how healed a state we reach, trauma might come up again. "That doesn't mean you're not healed," Lexi says. "It doesn't mean the work you did didn't matter. It just means that this is what's up for you today." She points out that all that past healing work means you're better qualified to handle what's coming up. You can regulate your emotions more smoothly and ask for support better. She says, "I just wish there was more gentleness around that because it's not a linear process." Sometimes we experience setbacks immediately after an assault, and sometimes issues come up years, even decades, later.

As a somatics coach, Lexi doesn't see her work as healing wounds. Rather, it's about trying to expand the resiliency of our nervous system and what we're capable of holding. Anything that feels big, or scary, is often arising out of our nervous system, which can run the whole show without our awareness. A lot of the time it's our body, not our mind, that's running the show. Lexi describes how being triggered is akin to pulling a rubber band as far as it's able to stretch, all the way to the edge. Asking anybody to hold that all the time would be immensely stressful. But if you start with a loose rubber band and slowly begin to stretch it, you can observe how it feels at each step. Working slowly, we can build more rebound capacity. Lexi says that triggers don't become easier. But once we build the muscles around handling difficult triggers, we're stronger. Being vulnerable doesn't become any easier, either—we just feel more comfortable doing it because we're more used to doing it. When new or long dormant triggers arise years from now, we can flex that muscle we've built and grow our resiliency even further. When hard things happen, we can hold ourselves up.

Sometimes survivors experience difficulties soon after we are assaulted. After a friend raped Danika when she was twenty years old, she tried to block out the experience as if it had never happened. Then she started getting sick. Danika went to the doctor, who failed to explain her stomach symptoms, then went back, and back again a third time. On the third visit, they didn't ask her further questions, and handed her a pregnancy test. "I was fifteen weeks pregnant, almost four months," Danika says. When she called the attacker with the news, he dismissed her reality and insisted she keep the baby in the same breath. She had an abortion, which she describes as difficult to experience but ultimately a good choice for her.

Several years after she was raped, Danika got married and began trying for a child. Throughout the process of trying to get pregnant she had surgeries to remove uterine polyps and ovarian cysts. First they scraped her uterus to try to fix the issue, then they determined it was too scarred for pregnancy after that. Doctors told her she would never carry a pregnancy to term. She miscarried repeatedly. Sex, already made complicated by her trauma history, became associated with her fertility issues and the accompanying emotional pain. Throughout the process, Danika felt besieged by guilt over the abortion she'd had after getting pregnant from rape years before, thinking "I had my chance and I blew it." She believed she was to blame for the reproductive difficulties. After years of keeping him in the dark, she finally told her husband about the assault. He didn't blame her and encouraged her to keep trying. Finally, she and husband successfully conceived.

But Danika spent the rest of her pregnancy terrified something would go wrong, like all the other times. But nine months later, she had a son. After her ordeal, Danika felt she had no reason to sleep with her husband anymore, and turned down every opportunity for sex. Thinking she was only fearful of another pregnancy, her husband got a vasectomy, but it didn't change anything; their relationship didn't become more sexual. She loved her husband, but after the birth of their son, they "very quickly just became best friends." They didn't pursue any type of couple's therapy. Danika assumed she had a naturally low libido and didn't think too much about the source of her sexual disinterest. Occasionally she had sex with her husband out of a sense of duty, but usually they didn't have sex at all.

Danika's husband was a great father and her best friend, and while the relationship wasn't under duress—neither party was talking about breaking up—Danika knew the mismatch in libido couldn't be making her partner happy. She decided they should try opening their relationship, at least on his end: he could have sex-only affairs while away on business trips. She had worked with somebody in an open relationship for two decades, so she had a role model for how it worked. She thought, "Well, that's progressive and smart, and I'm progressive and smart. Let's do that." Her husband agreed. She thinks, looking back, that he was grateful. Danika told him "It would be worse to me to find out you were lying." She cautioned, "Don't bring it home." He was ordered to tell her only what she asked.

Her husband went on a business trip not long after that conversation. Three weeks later, he returned home and sat Danika down to talk. "I met somebody," he said, "I'm in love, and I'm leaving you." Shocked, she couldn't believe that this was a possible outcome of their new agreement. Three weeks was all it took for him to become so attached to somebody else that he would blow up their entire life? "We had a deal," she recalls thinking. "We had ground rules."

Her husband left her for the woman he met while away on business. They got married, had two kids, and sixteen years later they're still together. "That was brutal," Danika tells me. Those experiences got her into counseling, specifically exploring what was going on with her low libido. It turned out it wasn't really low libido—it was "brain, mind, emotion stuff" related to the assault and its aftermath. Like many other survivors, it took a second difficult experience to get Danika into therapy and take on her trauma.

For Leanna, like many survivors, the years immediately following her sexual assault were marked by turmoil, issue after issue piling up. Right when she was getting into a healthy relationship with a new guy post-assault, she became unexpectedly pregnant.

Leanna was already struggling to cope with everyday life after the sexual assault. She realized her assault trauma as well as ongoing family issues could potentially affect her child, and she didn't think she would be able to handle raising a kid with her brand new partner. Plus, in order to make it work financially, she and her partner would have had to move back in with her parents, which would have exacerbated her trauma. All these factors played into her decision to put her daughter up for adoption.

Leanna is sad about the adoption to this day, but believes it was the right decision. Her daughter inspires her to make a better life for herself. Plus, she believes if she hadn't gotten pregnant she wouldn't have realized she needed to get her life together or be as far along in recovery as she is now.

I ask Leanna about her experience as a birth mother, explaining that to me, going through something new can inform your understanding of something that happened a long time ago, kind of like how a kaleidoscope has multiple intersecting prisms that shift as you move them.

Leanna explains that it was being a birth mom, not sexual assault, that ultimately got her into therapy. Her therapist, who she accessed through the adoption agency, reminded her of the original reason she ended up putting her daughter up for adoption: trauma from the assault. In therapy she dealt with postpartum hormonal changes and previously unaddressed PTSD at the same time, as well as the depression and upheaval inherent in the adoption process. Ultimately, she switched to a more trauma-centered therapist several months later. Leanna feels that until she started dealing with the sexual trauma in therapy, she was never able to put healthy distance between herself and the trauma. They talked through foundational survival skills, and a year or two later she was working on accepting and learning from her experience.

Leanna's partner was struggling with mental illness at the time, so they navigated their issues individually, not just together. As a couple, they learned that their sex life was tied inextricably to their mental health. They have an understanding that if one of them is having a rough time, sex might be off the table, or they could try something less intense, which for them looks like making out or oral sex. To Leanna, a trauma reaction intersects with her sex life particularly around intimacy. If she feels she can't connect with her own body, or is dissociating a lot, sex won't be a healthy choice for her. Both Leanna and her partner have leaned into the idea that saying no to each other can actually help their relationship grow. For survivors, setting boundaries around what we don't want can actually build space in which we feel more comfortable saying yes. It took a huge life upheaval to get Leanna on a healthy course, but that setback ultimately set her up for growth. While something may feel negative in the moment, learning from it and leaning into the growth process can lead to more positive sexual and relational outcomes in the future.

Leanna's experience reminds me of others who have become pregnant either as a result of rape or soon after their assault. The hormonal changes and physical nature of the pregnancy coupled with sexual trauma are enormously difficult. Other medical consequences of sexual assault can compound the trauma we experience.

Thirty years after she was raped, Danika was hospitalized. It turned out she had gotten herpes from the rape, and decades later the virus spread to her brain causing meningitis, an inflammation of the membranes that protect the brain. She had to have multiple medical procedures to deal with the fallout of the rape, decades later. However, Danika tells me she did not have to deal with stigma from the medical team that treated her meningitis. Perhaps, given the decades in between the rape and the diagnosis, the stigma some survivors face when seeking treatment for STDs was not there.

After a man raped my friend, she struggled to recover from the injuries for weeks. She was too in shock to go get STI-tested, and when she finally sought medical attention, it turned out that not only did she have more injuries than she had been aware of, but an STI, too. Luckily, it was curable with medication, but having been raised to believe STIs were a reflection of her moral value, she felt deeply ashamed about having contracted an illness from rape—even though it had nothing to do with her choices.

Since my friend fully recovered with medication, she doesn't have the burden of telling later partners about a challenging STI status or explaining that it came from a rape—but many people do. It becomes part of how we disclose our history to partners. For survivors who haven't been tested for STIs, doing so can be scary, but it's a necessary part of consent and open communication moving forward. No matter your STI status, or your medical history, none of us need more shame piled onto what our culture already tells us to feel.

Meningitis was not the only physical fallout of trauma Danika experienced. Danika's experience of the impact of sexual assault is very embodied. Throughout her adult life she had to deal with cysts on her ovaries and other growths, which she feels represent emotional difficulty she is burdened with. Navigating these physical issues has been made complicated by other problems, related to pain and sex, that stemmed from trauma. One doctor recommended a procedure on her uterus, which other women told her could make sex painful. Danika, having worked so hard to earn back her connection to pleasure, told the doctor no. Medical decisions can be complicated after sexual assault as survivors navigate embodied symptoms of trauma and shifting goals.

Sometimes, sexual trauma may impact us decades into the future. Our lives may look completely different than they did at the time of the assault, but trauma finds its way into our new relationships and day-to-day experience.

Years after she was assaulted, Laura moved back home and resumed her old job. She started dating a man from her past, and eventually they got married. Laura felt that, as a woman in her forties, kids were "icing on the cake" and not integral to the relationship—but her husband felt differently, and insisted they have kids together. This proved triggering to Laura in a new way, because where sex used to be a choice made by two individuals, it now became about a goal—reproduction. She didn't necessarily want to be having sex when she was ovulating and she reflects, "I think, for somebody who hasn't been raped, it might be different." She felt anger and frustration toward her new husband, who she felt was acting manipulatively. While Laura didn't like what was happening, she believed her husband deserved to be in a relationship with somebody who wanted to have sex with him, and she felt constantly conflicted.

Laura and her husband eventually had two kids, but their sexual issues didn't stop there. After having kids, her husband became irritated by her for not responding to his sexual advances the way he wanted. He called her a prude, and told her nine out of ten women wouldn't have a problem doing the things he wanted to do. Laura identifies as more vanilla than her husband and wants sex to be over quicker than he does. Over the years she has tried to "meet his needs because I just needed to . . . 'keep the household happy.'" She felt obligated to improve her husband's mood. But unwanted sex, to her, even if it's not violent, becomes triggering. He pressured her to perform, and when she pointed out that this made her feel bad, he became angry. One night, Laura's husband suggested they massage each other and then have sex. She responded, "Well, that's kind of two different things for me. Massage is relaxing, and I just want to chill after a massage. I don't feel like performing." That idea of "performing" slipped out, and her husband became upset, contesting the idea that she was putting on a show for him. "It is performing for me," Laura insisted. "Sometimes I'm doing it because I love you, and I want to make you happy, and not because I want to." Laura feels that her experience as a sexual assault survivor makes these issues more complex. We have to counter the narrative that our performance for partners is more important than our internal experience during sex. Being fulfilled by our experiences is often more aligned with our values than putting on a show for someone else.

Laura wishes people could talk more openly about sex and trauma, the way people seem willing to talk more openly about other personal issues, even somewhere public, like at a cocktail party. "We wouldn't feel the shame," Laura says, "and we wouldn't feel guilty for not giving sex to people who may love us, but want more sex than we want, and somehow we have to defer to their level of desire." Laura's needs and wants are different from her husband's, but instead of bending to his will, Laura stays centered in what she wants. It's not just about standing up for herself to her husband, but also in recognition of how her needs and wants have changed over time. "My terms are my terms," Laura says, "and I don't know what my terms are, because I'm entering a whole new stage of life." Staying open to changes in our own sexuality, even when our lives or sex lives become more challenging, allows us the freedom to explore what we want and need from ourselves and others.

Lexi spent a decade of her life post-assault taking apart the messages she received growing up and as a young adult that got in the way of her growth toward a fulfilling sexual and romantic life. While some aspects of her identity—like having autism and ADHD, veering toward people pleasing, and issues with autonomy—were somewhat more specific to her, Lexi identified one area that always set her back and many other people could identify with: breakups.

Even with poor or even harmful partners, Lexi never wants to hurt anybody during a breakup. Part of this, she feels, is a gendered pressure not to make anybody uncomfortable—including by breaking up with them, even if she's unhappy in the relationship.

Lexi points to the Disney movies she watched growing up to explain where some of this came from. In those films, characters magically developed relationships without ever having a single difficult conversation. "It's like we got in a fight," Lexi describes, "and we didn't talk for six months. And then we ran into each other at a flower market and just got back together." Lexi remembers questioning the characters' relationship: Where did they solve the problem? She tells me she never had cultural role models of women having difficult conversations or standing up for their needs.

Lexi grew up socialized with the idea that marriage is for life and relationships are for marriage. So, she felt pressured to create long-lasting relationships, even if the person she was with wasn't somebody she felt particularly aligned with. If she had feelings for them, that should be enough to maintain a long-term relationship. Lexi thought that you had to absolutely loathe your partner to actually break up with them.

As an adult, she began to unlearn this paradigm. Love alone wasn't enough to keep a relationship going. Most relationships, in Lexi's view, end when practical issues can't be overcome. She tells me she finds it difficult to feel justified in leaving a relationship. Lexi learned this while breaking up with a man who she dated for eight years, after getting together when she was twenty-two.

Looking back, she feels the power differential was too much to handle at twenty-two years old. He was a cuck, and wanted her to sleep with other people. After her trauma, Lexi struggled to sleep with new men and didn't want to do it. She felt pressured to act out her partner's fantasy: that she was his personal porn star. She in particular didn't like that he was selecting partners for her to sleep with who had bigger penises, which made her physically uncomfortable on top of being overall apprehensive about the encounters. Lexi didn't like sleeping with random men without any kind of connection, but that's what her partner wanted. Ultimately, she leaned on alcohol and substances to get to a mental place where she could manage sexual encounters with new partners. Over the years, she felt her primary partner was never pleased—if she refused to sleep with somebody else, he became angry, and if she did sleep with somebody, he would end up mad, too. There was no way to win.

Her post-assault relationship had a plus side: Lexi liked the power shift in her direction. As the only one having sex outside her relationship, she was in a more dominant role than she'd previously experienced with men. This dynamic proved healing to Lexi. However, while she was in control of her relationship with her partner, she still ended up drinking, contorting herself mentally to sleep with other people with whom she wasn't actually comfortable.

Finally, she felt she had poured so much energy into trying to make the relationship work that she was left totally burned out and unable to mask her autism and ADHD symptoms. Lexi's social orientation around pleasing a male partner was exacerbated by her trauma history and her desire to mitigate potential disagreement (and violence), as well as to give in to what a man wanted because that was the familiar dynamic. The night before her thirtieth birthday, she and her partner were in couple's therapy, and Lexi realized she just wanted to end it. Her attempt to break up with him in a respectful way devolved into messy conflict, and her ex became mean and cruel.

Looking back, Lexi feels like she did everything possible to preserve the relationship, but in the end, her ex hated her anyway. This proved difficult for someone socialized to believe her value was based on how others perceived her, especially men. But we don't get to control people's actions or reactions, Lexi points out. It's impossible to fully people please, because we're doing what we think somebody wants, not necessarily what they actually want. It's much healthier, Lexi thinks, "to be honest, to share honestly, and to ask honestly." Lexi had trouble ending that relationship because of her socialization around what she owed others, particularly men, and she grew from the experience, rethinking how relationships and breakups function.

Lexi explains that for trauma survivors, people pleasing can become a coping mechanism to try to minimize violence or pain. "I feel like so many of us are focused on not wanting to hurt other people," Lexi says, "that we aren't listening to what we want: Is this relationship working?" Lexi recalls her therapist telling her that the honeymoon period in a relationship can be any length of time, but is always "how long it lasts until the two people get into their very first conflict that is serious enough to end the relationship, but doesn't." Lexi acknowledges that a relationship has to involve love, but it has to function too. Questioning whether a relationship can function allows us to form solutions to problems that might arise.

Sometimes, romantic relationships aren't meant to stay romantic, but that doesn't necessarily mean a total social break needs to happen. If two people love each other but don't work well together, they can stay in each other's lives—what Lexi's current partner has done with an ex. Acknowledging how the relationship didn't function—in this case, her current partner and his ex were both avoidant and would go weeks without seeing each other—made space for them to stay friends, because they were grounded in reality. Lexi thinks it's important that the people she sees are committed to having vulnerable conversations together. At the end of the day, she wants to be on the same team, working toward the same goal, with somebody as honest as she is.

While it was difficult for her to break up with her ex, Lexi also sees breakups from the lens of the partner being broken up with. While many people say ghosting is mean and pressure people not to ghost their partners, she doesn't see people talking about how you can make it feel safe for others to tell you they're not interested. Lexi feels we don't have that cultural conversation going about dating and communication in relationships, new or long-standing. Lexi has observed friends and partners, reluctant to break up the way she used to be, afraid of becoming the villain in someone else's story. She tells me, we never want to be the bad guy—but we can't control other people's behavior. All we can do is show up with integrity and be true to ourselves.

Sexual assault survivors may experience medical setbacks from existing or new conditions made more difficult to manage because of trauma. In her twenties, Mia had her first bipolar episode. For that whole summer, she experienced hypersexuality. She had one physical drive—hypomanic hypersexuality—directly in conflict with her trauma response to shut down in sexual situations. Instead of ignoring sexual interest how trauma told her to, she acted impulsively. Her only saving grace, she says, was that she had a roommate keeping track of her comings and goings, or else she would've been out all night, every night. Her bipolar symptoms overpowered her trauma avoidance and while hypomanic, her focus was on the pursuit of sex. Mia feels like at her highest mood, she is "boisterous, hyperactive—always doing something, always talking to somebody. There's always something going on." When she feels depressed, she becomes convinced people don't want to hear from her, asking herself, "Why would they want to hear from me? I don't have anything to contribute." This feeling leads to social isolation, which becomes part of a cycle of low self-worth, reinforcing negative messages that she originally received from trauma.

Like Mia, I am bipolar. I've experienced episodes, from severe depression to mania, since I was fifteen years old. When it comes to sex and relationships, being bipolar has had a significant impact during mood episodes and even in the maintenance phase. When I'm depressed, I lose most feelings of attraction to other people—even people I know I like, or people who I can tell would be attractive to me if I was doing better. When manic, I experience hypersexuality, the medical term for heightened sex drive and a tendency to have riskier sex (meaning, in my case, sleeping with people I don't know well, having sex in uncertain environments, or not using condoms with people I don't know). During mixed episodes, when I experience symptoms of depression and mania, I may be driven by anger and irritability to find relief through sex, or have a high sex drive but feel less sensation or less attraction than I expect, a frustrating experience in its own right. And even when stable, medications I've taken affect things like my sleep drive or energy level, making it hard to date or sleep with people. All of this is made more difficult by the feeling that I "should" or "shouldn't" communicate what I'm feeling, going through, or dealing with in the moment. Often I end up having to make a double disclosure in order to feel comfortable: I have a history of trauma that affects sex and a mental illness that adds another layer of complexity.

As with reactions to my disclosure of my trauma history, partners' reactions to my mental illness run the gamut. Sometimes their responses are supportive and they ask how they can help. Sometimes the word "bipolar" sounds like a red flag to them, or they feel overwhelmed and don't have a positive response. A lot of people either minimize the severity of the illness, trying to write it off as akin to low-level depression, or it becomes a significant turnoff. Much of the time, I end up feeling like "a lot," like I'm too much for somebody new to handle no matter how much they like me or want to sleep with me. I find that when I don't disclose my mental illness, anything beyond a one-night stand becomes stressful. I feel like I'm lying. Much of the time, somebody's response to my condition has more to do with their previous exposure (or lack thereof) to other people who have a bipolar diagnosis. How they navigate our interaction is as affected by their history as my history affects the interaction, too.

When it comes to facing difficulties after sexual assault that intensify or change our trauma reactions, there's one issue that universally proves difficult: experiencing another assault. However, revictimization is common among survivors, and we can't have a conversation about healing from sexual assault without acknowledging the reality that some survivors are assaulted again. It's out of our control and terrible, but something we would do better to face than ignore.

Experiencing trauma doesn't act as a talisman against future pain; survivors are statistically more likely to be revictimized a second time.[1]

After a close friend heard I had been assaulted for a second time, he asked, in shock, "How could you of all people have this happen to you again?" He was referring to the fact that I had made a career out of helping people through trauma, and was aware of the great cost of trauma—how did I end up mired back in it again? His response hurt my feelings, but in a way I shared his perspective. Orienting my life away from assault hadn't protected me from it happening again. But that's the thing—assault has nothing to do with the victim's actions or intentions.

Decades after Ignacio was first sexually assaulted, their colleague turned what started out as a consensual hookup into a sexual assault. Ignacio had been lonely for a long time and agreed to play with their colleague with certain boundaries laid out clearly beforehand. After those boundaries were broken and the colleague sexually violated Ignacio, they felt completely silenced. They reverted back to not being able to speak and fell into a deep, suicidal depression. The shame they felt morphed into anger and self-blame, thinking it was their "bad decision" and loneliness that caused their emotional distress. Ignacio realized they needed to seek outside help to make it through, and put themself into a thirty-day recovery program. They realized they needed to talk about what happened, so they reached out and told friends what happened. Ignacio tells me, "When that happened, something inside of me said, 'You better tell somebody, you gotta talk. You gotta tell somebody,' . . . and so I did." Those conversations proved difficult, because Ignacio still blamed themself. They came up with a way of introducing the conversation to potential allies: "I need to talk to you about something, and I just need you to listen because I don't even know what I'm thinking here." Framing the crisis as something they were still working through helped them access supportive conversations with friends who may have otherwise reacted in a way that would not prove as helpful.

Thinking about what happened as "sexual assault," especially with their prior history of sexual assault, was difficult, so Ignacio focused on the way they were feeling instead of the legal language. They felt horrible, reflecting that they'd spent decades healing only to end up in a hurt position once again. Then it hit Ignacio: people feel like they've reached a point where they've healed, but things will still happen: "We can't control what people do. I have control over what I do." After that, rather than beating themself up, Ignacio shifted their focus to all the tools they were gaining through the experience they were going through. They reassessed their safety protocols around pickup play and how to talk to potential partners. They became more secure in their ground rules and boundaries for sexual encounters, as well as strategies they could use to get out of a bad situation in the moment. Learning from the assault and its aftermath helped Ignacio through.

It took several months for Ignacio to fully crawl out of the suicidal despair they fell into after being assaulted again. In the process, Ignacio connected with many friends and people in their life that had experienced additional trauma who showed up for them. Looking back, Ignacio feels a lot of empathy for the self-blaming version of themself that had to endure so much. They recognize that their agency was taken away from them, and while they had chosen to be alone with the person that assaulted them, they hadn't chosen to be assaulted. "It's a practice of being kind to myself when I make mistakes, because I am human," Ignacio says, "and I will continue to make mistakes until the day I die." They couldn't treat themself poorly every time they made one small choice that led to pain, or else they'd be in a state of suicidal ideation in perpetuity. Self-blame had to turn into patient self-compassion for Ignacio to survive, and return to their work helping other survivors and marginalized people.

Some survivors spoke about a second (or third) assault, and how it affected them. Others, like Mason, talked about negative sexual experiences that they wouldn't term assault, but which had a bad impact on them.

A couple of years before we spoke, Mason spent Thanksgiving alone not long after a breakup with his serious girlfriend of four years. He was struggling with everything, feeling bad about himself constantly. He "was not having any luck on the dating apps, at all." Thanksgiving Day hit, and Mason went on Grindr. He messaged with somebody and felt like they could have a fun encounter—it had been a while since he'd been touched and felt human. He felt good about the plan.

Mason went over to his hookup's house and hit the ring camera doorbell. The man he was meeting unlocked the door from his phone and told Mason to come join him upstairs where he was waiting for him, naked. "As soon as I saw him," Mason says, "I was like, that is not the person from the photos." He had shared a completely different person's photos to get Mason to come over. Mason remembers thinking, *I'm having a bad day, fuck it. This might as well happen, I don't care.* The man asked Mason to give him a blowjob. He got aggressive about it, "throat fucking [me] pretty hard . . . at the wrong angle." After the man finished, he said he wasn't in the mood to reciprocate. Soon, Mason was driving home, feeling incredibly low. On the drive, he questioned his choices that night, why he went over to the man's house, why he put up with the rough, one-sided encounter. Layered over his existing depression about losing his girlfriend, then having this terrible experience on Thanksgiving, a family holiday, Mason was left feeling more alone than ever.

Mason has ADHD, which is a condition that causes his body to produce too little dopamine. He finds he gets depressive episodes tied to that diagnosis. In combination with circumstantial depression from his partner leaving him, the breakup, and how his life was falling apart, he felt disconnected from everybody, including his family. "It was a perfect storm of stuff . . . calling back to trauma and shame and feeling like I don't have a place anymore." Twenty-five years after the trauma, the shame spiral he felt starting as a kid got whipped up into suicidality. It took a lot for Mason to unpack that bad hookup and what it meant for him moving forward. He has grown to value community and loving bonds with friends and lovers alike as a way to remedy the intense isolation he felt.

Sexual assault involves weaponizing somebody's sexuality, not interacting with someone consensually, Stacey points out. She emphasizes that consensual sex and sexual assault are not in the same category, and regretting something you do consensually isn't the same. If you retain agency during sex but don't like it and choose to continue it, that might be sex you regret; if your agency is taken from you and you can't choose to stop or keep going, if it's out of your hands, that is clear-cut sexual assault.

Maintaining that critical distance can be difficult, especially when microaggressions or assaults are being perpetrated by partners. Ramona views all her sexual interactions through a critical lens, and makes a practice of both noticing and sharing when something feels or felt off about a sexual encounter. It's challenging for her to express boundaries, and while she feels more comfortable with a person she's dating, she notices herself going along with hookups because she's worried she'll be viewed negatively for saying no. She isn't speaking so much about dangerous situations, but times that she ends up regretting doing something simply because she went along with it for the wrong reasons. She finds it's helpful to at least communicate more clearly afterward. "Maybe even if I wasn't able to say in the moment that something was bothering me, [I'll] send a text the day after," explaining how she felt. She might acknowledge that they didn't mean to do anything wrong, and go on to explain that the end result was not okay with her.

Ramona has a strong sense of boundaries. Even dating while in high school, she felt pretty decisive and communicative. She noticed whenever that wasn't being fully respected, and her consciousness around her boundaries helped her navigate dating even at that early age. After the #MeToo movement became popular, Ramona has noticed men have been more open to receiving those conversations. She has noticed that trauma responses can get in the way of communication when it comes to sexual boundaries, but at this point she has over a decade of practice in laying down boundaries and reinforcing them later on.

Another survivor friend of mine who had been assaulted by somebody she was dating later experienced the end of a different relationship because of lying and cheating. She told me how bad it felt to work hard to trust somebody, only to have them turn around and hurt her. Even though the breakdown in trust happened for a different reason—cheating—she felt a familiar type of devastation. It brought up some of the same emotions and thought patterns as her assault. In order to move forward, she had to work through some of her old emotional responses and issues with trust. It felt like going back in time, like being caught in an endless cycle of pain.

I ask Lyndsey how she ended up with her husband, after a slew of negative dating experiences post-assault. She explains that soon into their relationship, she strongly considered breaking up with him, despite their connection and her newfound confidence in herself, because "it's hard to be with someone who just genuinely likes you." He did not pressure her for sex, loved her dog, and sharing responsibilities in her life, from the jump. It was her first meaningful exposure to somebody who liked her so much, and the dissonance caused her trauma brain to kick in and try to push him away. "The only reason I didn't," Lyndsey says, "is because I was still in therapy." Her therapist told her the relationship was actually good for her, and she didn't have to run away from a positive influence. Lyndsey was resistant, explaining, "The closer you get to a good thing—that's when you could really get hurt." She felt it was all too good to be true, and terrified that she might experience further emotional pain by trusting her new partner and giving their relationship her all. But she stayed, and he proved over and over again that he really did care about her. She ultimately accepted that she could have a good relationship, and today, they are married.

After the first time a man raped me, I was so focused on finding somebody—anybody—that could handle my trauma within a romantic and sexual relationship that I lost my focus on what other factors mattered. Years later, after another assault and breakup, I decided to explore beyond those specific checkboxes. What else was out there?

I decided to collect some data by going on a slew of dates and sleeping around more intentionally, almost like an experiment. I slept with people I didn't know, and new friends. I didn't disclose much of my trauma history—though my work on the issue usually meant I talked about it in some capacity—and I was more interested in exploring what different matches could yield in terms of a sexual dynamic I genuinely enjoyed, beyond that baseline "handles trauma well" factor. I found several people who handled trauma poorly, for their own reasons, and others who I enjoyed sleeping with once I'd established enough of a sense of safety that I was comfortable exploring.

The setback of the second assault on top of the life-disrupting breakup could have caused me to shut down, but instead, I opened up. I found myself working out old issues related to trauma by exploring new dynamics with new people. I tested out whether it felt bad if somebody pushed my boundaries—or if I'd developed enough trust with them that I knew they would respect a hard "no." I allowed partners to take the reins in a way I'd always avoided, afraid to lose control in case trauma took over.

In many ways, sex with semi-strangers proved distracting, almost a form of pain relief, in a way that most other activities couldn't, because it engaged the side of my brain tied up in trauma, too. I was always spending time with my trauma, but when I went out and slept with people, that time wasn't triggering—it was healing. Slutty phases, as my friends and I call them, can be reactionary to something bad, like trauma, but in this case, I was determined to harness my curiosity and grow. I decided to phoenix myself out of a situation I'd hoped never to find myself in again. Early one morning, just after a man left my house after we slept together, I went out on my porch with my dog. My body felt stretched and sore, tired and very alive. I gave myself a high five for being brave with this new person, putting myself out there despite recent pain. I also couldn't stop grinning, the residue of pleasure sticky on my skin. I probably wasn't going to sleep with this guy again, I knew. But I found meaning in the interaction because of what it meant for myself: Unlike after the previous assault, I wasn't stuck. I was growing.

After the better part of a year of this, I got tired of constantly starting over with new people, and settled toward a middle ground: unafraid to try on someone new, but more interested in seeing where things could actually end up with the right person. I'm still searching, still growing, and still open to what comes next.

Aftercare:
The Future of Sex

A LISA LEARNED ABOUT aftercare from friends in the kink community. She explains, "We all might need different things, or just simply want different things in the aftermath of a sexual experience, especially if that experience is newer to us or more experimental to us." One of the first times she thought about what her aftercare needs were was at the beginning of her current relationship. It was long distance, and she realized she didn't want to have sex and then feel like she or her partner were immediately about to leave for the airport. She realized this was actually an aspect of aftercare: She needed to be physically present with the person she slept with for twenty-four hours after they had sex. Being physically present was tied to feeling stability, comfort, and a continuation of intimacy so that it wasn't cut off the moment after sex ended.

While her current partner offers the stability of aftercare from another person, Alisa had to learn to practice her own aftercare when she was single, because partners weren't necessarily providing everything she needed. To her, aftercare can mean a wide range of behaviors, from debriefing with a post-sex conversation—not just what happened, but also how it made her feel—or having her partner make her a sandwich and hang out for a while, or smoking a joint, taking a nap: to her, the activity didn't necessarily have to specifically matter. Connection post-sex was the key.

The last person I interviewed for this book was Ignacio, whose life work centered around issues related to this book. Toward the end of our interview, in one of the most steadying experiences of the previous few months of my life, I became honest with them, explaining that I moved to my current city less than a year before. I'd been trying to make new friends and build a social life. I explained, "I've been sleeping with sluts, but I have not made slutty friends, and nobody will really engage with me in these conversations. So sometimes when I talk to people for the book, it's the first time in a couple of weeks where I had a good conversation." Sleeping with people who were sexually open-minded wasn't the same as having a community of people to *talk to* about doing that. It wasn't until I started having conversations like the ones recorded in this book that I felt supported in my sexual exploration. Without intending to, research for this book proved to be as normalizing for me as I hope the book itself will be for others.

Social support is the biggest predictor of healing trauma, whether that's support from a partner, a friend, or a community that recognizes a survivor's pain and needs moving forward.[2] Often, in our quest to reclaim our sexuality and regain a sexual sense of self, we feel isolated. Our culture tells us that sex is something that happens behind closed doors, and we should keep our healing process to ourselves, or talk about it only with our partners. The truth is, all of us would benefit from swapping stories with other survivors, from having people hear us, from having somewhere to go when our partner isn't available, or when we don't have one.

One morning while deep into research, I got on a Zoom call with a survivor I'd previously interviewed, Leanna. As she spoke, I found myself thinking about the man who I'd had over the night before, Gabriel. He was a casual partner—the one so good at embodied consent—and I wasn't expecting to hear from him particularly soon, but something was on my mind. I'd seen Gabriel three times thus far, and he'd always become uncomfortable when I brought up my trauma history or talked about how trauma impacted sex. His hesitancy and resistance to listening well made those conversations feel like pulling teeth. In order to move forward with him, those conversations felt necessary to me.

I ask Leanna if I can tell her about something from my own life, switching the spotlight from her to me. She says sure. Reflecting on disclosing some of my trauma history to Gabriel, I tell her, "I was like, 'How have you not had some version of this conversation before?'" Leanna agrees and points out that people need to be made to feel comfortable sharing things, and not have the "what the fuck Pikachu face" thrown at them. Don't say "What the hell are you talking about?" or "Why would you say this to me?" Talking to Leanna, a survivor with insight into the exact phenomenon I was describing, about something happening in real time, made me feel so much less alone. I also realized that even years after I was assaulted, I often still feel like I'm supposed to be returning to some healthy starting point, to hit reset—but really, what I'm most craving is people to heal with throughout my journey. Even later, reading the transcript of my conversation with Leanna, it makes me feel more normal. It's my goal for every person reading this to have a moment like mine, or many, when we go from feeling strange for wanting what we want, to feeling held.

Sometimes I showed up on Zoom a few hours after somebody I liked or slept with had left my house. Without directly asking those interviewees about whatever was bothering me from the previous night, I would gain insight into my own experience through our conversations. I was looking for answers for other people, but I found them for myself, too. Whether it was Leanna describing how surprises during sex, even positive ones, feel bad in her body, or Mason explaining that pleasure focused only on him made him uncomfortable, or Alisa pointing out that we owe our partners the same opportunity to set boundaries with us as we want from them, I saw myself in these sexual assault survivors' stories, and more often than not, I learned something from them that I carry with me to this day.

As I researched and wrote this book, I changed. I gained life experience related to relationships, sex, and trauma, that impacted the questions I asked of survivors and the way I formulated my own answers. Hearing so many perspectives and putting them in conversation with one another on the page, I reflected on what the future of sex looks like, not just for survivors, but for our culture as a whole. In a world in which sexual assault survivors are turned into numbers on a page, centering our own individual needs—whether that looks like what survivors in this book have described or not—is a radical act, and the only way forward. What we want as people matters more than any cultural rules we've been indoctrinated with. Consent requires our individual presence in the moment. We center our perspective in our own life experience and shift away from getting overly attached to any prewritten story about what happens next. All of our experiences are valid; all of our experiences should be normalized. We get to choose what we want for ourselves. If something doesn't work out for us, we can reach for the next person, the next experience, the next relationship, until we find what feels right for us.

Mia is a public defender, a job that requires her to empathize with perpetrators of violent crime—a job she's wanted for a very long time, and which she decided to continue pursuing, despite her history of assault. Mia says, "Someone raping me does not mean I can't do what I set out to do." Leanna, who has made enormous strides in her life post-trauma, has settled around her decision not to go out at night alone—potentially a form of avoidance, but for her, a middle ground she feels comfortable holding, for now. I came to terms with my gendered sexual history—mostly men, some women, a lot of shame—and decided to stop hiding behind the heteronormativity I had leaned on in early adulthood. Now, to everyone, I'm bi and nonbinary. For all survivors, though, what we need, what we want, and what we reject, will change over time. Maybe, in the future, Mia will switch to a new and different career, Leanna will stop avoiding that trigger, and the way I express and describe my sexuality will shift. The future of sex is the future; we cannot know what's coming.

It's also uncertain because it doesn't only depend on us. It depends just as much on our partners' wants and needs. It's about whether or not the people I want to sleep with want to sleep with me. Being comfortable with fluctuations in needs, desires, partners, and boundaries is what I want out of my sex life. The perspective about my own sex life and sexuality I put down in this book will likely have changed by the time it is published. Not only is that okay, in a way, that's actually the point. And—for me—maybe more important than any particular aspect of my sex life: I want people to talk to, to work through how assault continues to affect sex. I want community.

Alisa feels she was socialized to ignore her own need for aftercare, never speak up for herself, and not communicate about it. She tells me she felt pressured to act like she didn't care: "Don't be the person to bring up brunch. Don't be the girl who suggests the continuation of the hang after the night—he has to suggest it." The message was clear: don't communicate, don't have needs, even after you have sex. Those are today's dating norms, but as a sexual assault survivor, they didn't serve her. Learning about aftercare was in direct conflict with messages like that, messages she learned growing up. Alisa thinks that many people of any gender desire softness and tenderness after sex—in her words, "everyone deserves to be spooned if they want to be spooned." When we connect with others over our needs related to sex, we are building the community I envisioned.

Aftercare is a powerful concept outside of sexual encounters. What does care look like for people who have experienced sexual trauma and are now healing? What can our communities, partners, therapists, loved ones do to better honor our needs post-assault? I have had a sexual encounter with a new partner that went poorly because of trauma, and felt like I had nobody to talk to about the experience. In those moments, I often wish I could speak more openly to not just my support network, but to the partner, too. And when things don't work out, I often mourn the loss of that person as a listening ear to talk about trauma and work through sexual issues. I used to write off ex-sexual partners, as modern dating rules require. Those people would no longer be a part of my healing journey. And then I met Solomon.

There are more outcomes than breakups or happily ever after endings—for relationships, and for people. While writing this book, I went on a couple of dates with a new friend. We had a lot in common, and I told him that talking to him felt like talking to myself, but there was somebody there to laugh at the jokes. Early on, I disclosed some of my trauma history, and he reacted exactly how I wish all partners would react: accepting my reality, asking what he could do to support me, and when roadblocks came up, like triggers during sex or different communication needs, he was patient and understanding that because of my history, those needs had to come first.

Ultimately, we did not develop a further sexual relationship, but decided to stay friends. As we got closer, I told him more about the distant, and more recent, trauma I was dealing with. Solomon turned quickly from a friend with benefits to a friend who helped me start the process of researching safety measures I could take—if I wanted—against somebody who had assaulted me. When I look at the security camera outside my front door, I recall Solomon putting it up. The closeness we cultivated through briefly going out and sleeping together translated into a relationship based on trust and empathy, and with Solomon's support, I felt able to take serious steps toward cultivating actual safety in my life—the safety I needed to move forward as a person, not just as somebody's sexual partner.

Solomon would never sleep over after we had sex, but later, after we became friends, I faced a crisis that threatened my immediate safety, and he spent the night in my bed. I remember waking up from a nightmare, the world still dark and a pillow between us. My hand reached for his back to steady me. In the morning, I felt stable enough to take the steps toward safety that had so paralyzed me the day before. Solomon had validated all my fears and reassured me that my strong reaction and emotional response was merited—in many ways, the opposite of perpetrators of violence I have experienced, who gaslit me and manipulated me into doing what *they* wanted. Simply sleeping next to him felt a lot like aftercare: spending time together in a soothing way, either sleeping or doing something relaxing, that allowed me to recenter myself in my own experience before I went back out into the world.

This relationship with Solomon gave me a powerful feeling of safety and protection, but it also led to changes within my own life and my perspective on what has happened to me. Solomon was quick to label abuse as abuse, while many other people I had known for longer were hesitant, maybe out of a desire to protect me from bad things. But those bad things had happened, Solomon always pointed out. As I talked with him more and as he showed up, repeatedly, to support me through a difficult time, I realized that maybe this is what many abuse victims actually need out of a relationship. We don't heal in a vacuum, we heal as we're moving through our lives: in my case, starting over in a state halfway across the country, rebuilding my social life from the ruins an abusive man had left it in, and trying to date and sleep with new people—all while writing an inherently triggering book. We need somebody to recognize not just our sexual needs, but our need for an actual, deep feeling of safety that isn't necessarily what a traditional relationship entails. Solomon and I didn't work out as sexual partners, but what he gave me was what most of us survivors need from partners: recognition of what happened to us and acceptance of the fact that our trauma may be the driving force behind what we need from a relationship, not a secondary consideration.

The reality is, we don't often run into the right person to meet our needs or our desires. Mason didn't find a partner who found his bisexuality hot, and his trauma worth caring about, until he was in his late thirties. Many of the older women I interviewed for this book didn't find the pleasure-focused sex they'd been unable to access, stuck in difficult marriages, for decades. Some survivors I spoke to appeared stuck even while we spoke: unable to articulate or prioritize their needs, or in the midst of life changes that precluded them from accessing their full sexuality, their full humanity. In those moments, tethered too far from those parts of ourselves, we may be tempted to abandon our sexual selves. But remarkable to me is how these survivors from all backgrounds at all stages of recovery and all stages of life, refused to give up. We can always choose to leave bad situations. We can always be patient, see where things go. We can always make changes. We can always choose ourselves.

There is a popular idea that somebody you sleep with will either turn into your life partner or disappear from your life completely. But when I consider the many stories shared in these pages, I think sexual assault survivors are shifting away from this paradigm. Instead of following prescribed ideas around what relationships can look like, we're approaching them with our particular needs front of mind. The partner of a sexual assault survivor may act differently from how a typical partner is expected to act. Sometimes we don't need sex—we need support. Sometimes, a survivor may be fresh out of an abusive relationship, or something brings a trigger front and center that they thought had been quelled long ago. I like to think of it like an acute injury that turns chronic. Supporting a survivor in the throes of fresh pain will look different from meeting the needs of a survivor who is years past an assault. Both survivors deserve sex and sexual partners that understand their needs, and are honest about whether they can meet them.

I like to think that if two potential partners come together and realize they won't work sexually, they could arrive at an understanding similar to what Solomon and I found: We didn't need to sleep together, but I did need help feeling safe—and actually building a safe life. I chose to meet some of Solomon's needs, too, mainly his need for close friendship from a like-minded person during a turbulent time in his life. Asking for your genuine needs is the only way to get them met. Even if we don't find the right person, we can keep looking to get our needs met outside of traditional romantic relationships: through loved ones, aid from organizations that care, love from pets, therapeutic relationships, hotlines, support groups, community gatherings, and even nature. For me, this radical reconceptualization of human needs is what post-traumatic growth looks like: being flexible in our understanding of our needs and the ways we might meet them, and brave enough to ask our partners, friends, and community for help in doing so. We are not alone.

Resources

For immediate assistance in case of an emergency, dial 911 or your local emergency services.

Help with Sexual Assault and Trauma

Suicide and Crisis Lifeline
https://988lifeline.org
Dial 988

National Domestic Violence Hotline
https://www.thehotline.org/
Dial 1-800-799-SAFE

WomensLaw: Legal help for abuse victims
https://www.womenslaw.org/

Veterans Affairs: Resources about PTSD
https://www.ptsd.va.gov/

National Sexual Violence Resource Center
https://www.nsvrc.org/

Planned Parenthood: Sexual health care
https://www.plannedparenthood.org/

The Trevor Project: For young LGBTQ+ survivors
https://www.thetrevorproject.org/

1in6: For male survivors
https://1in6.org/

Google "sexual assault help + [name of nearest city]" for more local options

To Find a Therapist

Psychology Today
https://www.psychologytoday.com/us/therapists/

BetterHelp
https://www.betterhelp.com/

Talkspace
https://www.talkspace.com/

For Sexuality and Sexual Health Information

Kinsey Institute: Sexuality and gender
https://kinseyinstitute.org/

OMGYES: Female pleasure
https://www.omgyes.com/

Planned Parenthood: Sexuality and sexual health
https://www.plannedparenthood.org/learn

Further Reading on Sexual Trauma and Sexuality

Speak by Laurie Halse Anderson
Our Bodies, Ourselves by Boston Women's Health Book Collective
Is Rape a Crime? by Michelle Bowdler
Ace by Angela Chen
The Ethical Slut by Dossie Easton and Janet Hardy
Not That Bad, edited by Roxane Gay
Healing Sex by Staci Haines
Trauma and Recovery by Judith Herman
Truth and Repair by Judith Herman
She Comes First by Ian Kerner
In the Dream House by Carmen Maria Machado
Know My Name by Chanel Miller
Crazy Love by Leslie Morgan
Come as You Are by Emily Nagoski
Come Together by Emily Nagoski
Mating in Captivity by Esther Perel
Want by Julie Peters
No Visible Bruises by Rachel Louise Snyder
Hot and Unbothered by Yana Tallon-Hicks
Sex Object by Jessica Valenti
Healing Honestly by Alisa Zipursky

Acknowledgments

THIS BOOK BEGAN as a series of interviews for a newspaper article I wrote when I was twenty-six years old. Seven years later, I am immeasurably grateful to the dozens of survivors whose stories made it into these pages. Your voices shine through on each page, and act like beacons in the night whenever I'm lost or struggling—and I'm sure you will help guide many others to their best sexual selves, too. And thank you to all the brave people, survivors or not, willing to talk about sex and sexual assault in the same sentence—we need your voices.

Thank you to *Tin House*, *Women's Health*, and the *Washington Post*, especially my editor Neema Roshania Patel, for publishing my early work on this hard-to-talk-about topic.

Thank you to Reiko Davis and DeFiore & Company, for your care for this project and its message, and our many exciting conversations about how to best connect this book with its audience. Thank you to Denise Silvestro and the team at Kensington Books, for giving me the opportunity to bring these stories to a broader audience.

Thank you to my early mentors and writing friends, especially teachers at Cabot Elementary School, Brown Middle School, Concord Academy, and later New York University, GrubStreet, University of East Anglia, and Columbia University: Penny Benjamin, Mr. Guerreio, Deanna Douglas, Jen Cardillo, June Foley, David Lipsky, Darrin Strauss, Ann Hood, Barbara Jones, Alex Marzano-Lesnevich, Amanda Petrusich, Allie Rowbottom, Garrard Conley ("Just try it!"), Sara Petersen, Iain Thompson, Kathryn Hughes, Helen Smith, Cailey Rizzo (for being fearlessly supportive of this project from day one), Jenessa Abrams and the Narrative Medicine innovators, and

Leslie Morgan (my trusted advisor on all things publishing). Thanks to Sarah Chaves for endless developmental feedback (on my book and myself) and to Pyae Moe Thet War, my most insightful cheerleader even several oceans away. And thanks to Christy, Caroline, Sam and Katie, Shayna, Miriam, Seth, David, and Will Levitt for your support and advice on confidence, marketing and publicity, and dating. Thanks also to the Kinsey Institute, for the sex ed dreams are made of.

Thank you to the queer and Jewish communities of Austin, where I have found friends and infinite title-brainstorming buddies. Thank you to my health-care team and to my ever-expanding rabbinate, for keeping me alive and in community. Thank you to the coffee shops and breweries around Austin where I camped out until I made my word count, and especially to Shalom Austin, my safehouse away from home.

Thank you to my family of origin: my parents, Patty and Dick, for letting me buy hardcover books and endless journals, then encouraging me to live a life to fill their pages; my brothers, Alex and Ben, for supporting me through the dark times and eating our way through the good times (and for adding fun people to the family, too!); Shirley Simon, my grandmother, a published author herself, for checking on my life as often as the lives I'm always writing about. Thank you to Lavonda, love of my life.

And to Babka, my best friend and the cutest possible reason to get up in the morning, who barked through every. single. interview. I promise we'll go to the park when I'm done editing this book.

Endnotes

Introduction

1. Rothbaum, Barbara Olasov, et al. "A Prospective Examination of Post-Traumatic Stress Disorder in Rape Victims." Wiley Online Library, John Wiley & Sons, 19 Feb. 2006. https://onlinelibrary.wiley.com/doi/10.1002/jts.2490050309.

Chapter 1

1. Dingfelder, S. F. "What Lies Behind the Female Habit of 'Tending and Befriending' During Stress." *Monitor on Psychology*, 35(1), January 1, 2004. https://www.apa.org/monitor/jan04/habit.
2. https://www.nhs.uk/mental-health/conditions/post-traumatic-stress-disorder-ptsd/complex/.

Chapter 2

1. "Victims of Sexual Violence: Statistics," RAINN, https://www.rainn.org/statistics/victims-sexual-violence.

Chapter 3

1. https://www.nhs.uk/mental-health/conditions/post-traumatic-stress-disorder-ptsd/symptoms/.
2. Herman, J., *Trauma and Recovery*, 1992, p. 8.
3. Maxfield, Louise, and Roger M. Solomon. "Eye Movement Desensitization and Reprocessing (EMDR) Therapy." American Psychological Association, 31 July 2017. www.apa.org/ptsd-guideline/treatments/eye-movement-reprocessing.

Chapter 5

1. Zemteno, S., Hilty, E., & Richard, K. (2023). Prevention is a team sport: Empowering male student athletes in your game place for campus sexual assault prevention. *It's on Us.*

Chapter 6

1. "Victims of Sexual Violence: Statistics," RAINN, https://www.rainn.org/statistics/victims-sexual-violence.
2. Abma, Joyce C., and Gladys M. Martinez, edited by Division of Vital Statistics, US Department of Health and Human Services, p. 5, "Sexual Activity and Contraceptive Use Among Teenagers in the United States," 2011–2015.

Chapter 7

1. https://www.law.cornell.edu/uscode/text/10/920#:~:text=7)%20 Consent.%E2%80%94-,(A),resistance%20does%20not%20constitute%20 consent.
2. https://www.plannedparenthood.org/learn/relationships/sexual-consent.
3. Brown, A. M., *Pleasure Activism: The Politics of Feeling Good*, AK Press, 2019, p. 15.

Chapter 8

1. "Post-Traumatic Stress Disorder," National Institute of Mental Health, U.S. Department of Health and Human Services, May 2019, www.nimh.nih.gov/health/topics/post-traumatic-stress-disorder-ptsd/index.shtml.
2. "Victims of Sexual Violence: Statistics," RAINN, www.rainn.org/statistics/victims-sexual-violence.
3. "APA Dictionary of Psychology: Trigger," American Psychological Association, dictionary.apa.org/trigger.
4. Sloan, Sara, PhD. "What's the Difference Between a Kink and a Fetish?" Mindbodygreen, 24 Apr. 2020, www.mindbodygreen.com/articles/kink-vs-fetish.
5. Malz, Wendy. "Moving Toward Healthy Sexual Behavior, Avenue 2: Take a Healing Vacation from Sex." *The Sexual Healing Journey: A Guide for Survivors of Sexual Abuse*, 3rd ed., Morrow, 2012, pp. 187–197.
6. Sagarin, Brad, "Never Tried BDSM? Go On, It's Good for You," *The Guardian*, Guardian News and Media, 9 Feb. 2015, www.theguardian.com/commentisfree/2015/feb/09/bdsm-good-for-you-fifty-shades-of-grey-relationship.
7. May, Gareth. "Your Brain on BDSM: Why Getting Spanked and Tied Up Makes You Feel High." *VICE*, 16 Feb. 2017, www.vice.com/en/article/j5e833/your-brain-on-bdsm-why-getting-spanked-and-tied-up-makes-you-feel-high.
8. Lorde, Audre, "Uses of the Erotic," *Your Silence Will Not Protect You*, Silver Press, 2017, p. 24.

9. Sauvageau, Anny, and Stéphanie Racette. "Autoerotic Deaths in the Literature from 1954 to 2004: A Review." *Journal of Forensic Sciences* 51.1 (2006): 140–146.

10. Hucker, S. J. "Sexual Masochism: Psychopathology and Theory," in *Sexual Deviance: Theory, Assessment, and Treatment*, D. R. Laws and W. T. O'Donohue, Eds. Guilford Press, New York, 1978, pp. 250–263.

11. "Everything You Need to Know About Erotic Asphyxiation," *Healthline*, Healthline Media, 29 May 2019, www.healthline.com/health/healthy-sex/erotic-asphyxiation#responsible-play.

12. Herman, Judith Lewis, "Disconnection," *Trauma and Recovery: The Aftermath of Violence—from Domestic Abuse to Political Terror*, Basic Books, 2015, p. 58.

13. Barrett-Ibarria, Sofia. "BSDM Can Provide Profound Healing Experiences." *VICE*, 29 Aug. 2017, https://www.vice.com/en/article/nee9yg/bsdm-can-provide-profound-healing-experiences.

14. Brown, A. M., "Introduction," *Pleasure Activism: The Politics of Feeling Good*, AK Press, 2019, p. 12.

15. Peters, Julie. "Step 5: Pleasure." *Want: 8 Steps to Recovering Desire, Passion, and Pleasure After Sexual Assault.* Mango Publishing Group, 2019, p. 126.

16. Glover, Cameron. "It's Time to Recenter Kink and BDSM as Part of Radical Queer History." *Slate*, 7 Nov. 2018, slate.com/human-interest/2018/11/kink-bdsm-radical-queer-history.html.

17. Easton, Dossie, and Janet W. Hardy. "Kink, Leather, and BDSM." *The Ethical Slut: A Practical Guide to Polyamory, Open Relationships and Other Freedoms in Sex and Love*, 3rd ed., Ten Speed Press, 2017, p. 42.

Chapter 9

1. https://www.researchgate.net/figure/The-average-duration-of-orgasm-10-12-Figure-3-above-indicates-the-average-duration-of_fig2_369093841#:~:text=Several%20researchers%20have%20reported%20the,minutes%20on%20average%20to%20orgasm.

Chapter 10

1. https://permanent.access.gpo.gov/gpo11287/216002.pdf.

2. Calhoun, C. D., Stone, K. J., Cobb, A. R., Patterson, M. W., Danielson, C. K., & Bendezú, J. J. (2022). "The Role of Social Support in Coping with Psychological Trauma: An Integrated Biopsychosocial Model for Posttraumatic Stress Recovery." *Psychiatric Quarterly*, 93(4), 949–970. https://doi.org/10.1007/s11126-022-10003-w.

Index

abortion, 190, 191
abusive relationships, 10–11, 15–30, 68, 74,
    102–103, 120, 122–123, 174, 213–216
activism, 20
acupuncture, 79
ADHD. *See* attention-deficit/hyperactivity
    disorder
adoption, 61–63, 192–193
adult playtime, 170–171
aftercare, 209–216
age differences, in relationships, 25–26
age play, 136–137, 165
alcohol use, 119, 143, 152, 198
Alexis (survivor), 20, 158–161
Alisa (survivor), 42–44, 51, 80–81, 83–84,
    108–110, 117, 137–138, 144–145,
    152–154, 163–164, 177–178, 181, 209,
    211, 213
anal sex, 126, 151
anniversary of sexual assault, 164
anxiety, 3, 63, 82, 148, 153, 162
apologies, 10, 22, 65, 143
appearance, value from, 49
arousal, during assault, 175
asexuality, 52–53, 96
attention-deficit/hyperactivity disorder
    (ADHD), 51, 66, 103–104, 196, 198,
    204
audio triggers, 93, 163
autism, 51, 66, 103–105, 196, 198
avoidance, 3, 36, 118, 152, 175, 199, 200, 212

BDSM. *See* bondage, discipline, dominance
    and submission, sadomasochism
BetterHelp, 218
binge eating, 48–49
bipolar disorder, 200–201
bisexual survivors. *See* LGBTQ+ survivors
blame, 43–44, 104, 125, 153, 191, 202, 203

Blonde (album), 71
Bloom, Danika (survivor), 13, 81–82, 102,
    119–120, 138–140, 182, 190–192, 194
blowjobs. *See* oral sex
bodily autonomy, 24, 34, 117, 148, 196
body
    connection of mind and, 128–129
    manifestation of trauma in, 12, 63
    reaction of, to triggers, 149, 152, 153, 156
    relationship with, 3, 48, 66, 74, 98–99
    sexualization of, 13
    trust in, 177, 179
body dysmorphia, 48
body image, 48–50
body language, 131–132, 141–143, 166
body scanning, 37
bodywork, 103. *See also* somatics
bondage, discipline, dominance and
    submission, sadomasochism (BDSM),
    14–15, 57, 124, 137, 151, 156–157, 160,
    162, 165–168
boundaries
    after setbacks, 203
    asserting, 14–15, 25, 30, 31, 37, 50–51, 53,
      64–66, 205
    consent and, 104, 132–135, 138
    disclosure and, 95–97, 100, 101, 109
    dismissing, 114
    enforcing, 138–139
    initial validation and adoption of, 170
    playing with, 134–137
    reinforcing, in kink community, 151–152
    respecting partners', 144–145, 211
    testing partners' respect for, 140–142
    tolerating violations of, 126–128
    and trauma-specific triggers, 154–155
    violating, 95–96
brainspotting, 75
breadcrumbing, 60

breakups, 4, 10–11, 17–21, 24–30, 74, 126–127, 174, 187–189, 196–200, 203–204, 206
brown, adrienne maree, 138, 163

casual sex (sleeping around), 2, 4, 10, 42–43, 103, 112, 119–120, 137–138, 142, 149–150, 152, 154–155, 159, 179–181, 206–208, 210–211. *See also* hookups; one-night stands
CBT (cognitive behavioral therapy), 63, 75
celibacy, 42, 43, 118, 124, 127–128, 152
cheating. *See* infidelity
checking in with yourself, 33–58
    about influences on behavior, 45–48
    on body image/identity issues, 48–54
    body scanning in somatics, 36–37
    getting caught up in others' perspectives vs., 33–35
    media representations and, 42–45
    and persistence of trauma, 35–36
    on sex education, 37–42, 54–58
childhood sexual abuse (CSA), 2, 4–5, 33, 40–42, 45–46, 58, 73, 108, 113, 117, 136, 137
choking, 134, 147, 158, 160–161
closeness, after disclosure, 100, 106
CNC (consensual nonconsent) sex, 78, 79
codependency, 66–67
coercion, 26
cognitive behavioral therapy (CBT), 63, 75
collaring, 134
communication, 67–68, 72, 75–76, 81, 83–85, 102–107, 112, 124, 127–128, 135, 137, 144, 148–150, 155, 157, 160, 165–170, 205, 213. *See also* disclosure of trauma history
compartmentalization, 16–17, 69, 94
complex post-traumatic stress disorder (C-PTSD), 9, 29–30, 82
connection, 184–186, 209, 213
consensual nonconsent (CNC) sex, 78, 79
consent, 1, 7, 131–146, 212
    in abusive relationships, 23, 25–27, 30
    and boundaries, 104, 132–135, 138
    controlling encounters with, 152
    defining, in reaction to assault, 138–140
    and disclosure, 104, 105
    dubious, 140
    embodied, 131–132, 137, 141–143, 165, 166, 210

gradual changes in, 139–140
    and healing through fantasies, 83–84
    in health-care setting, 177
    in kink and BDSM, 160, 162, 165, 166
    legal vs. functional, 132–133
    from partners, 142–146
    playing with, 134–137
    positive definition of, 133–134, 138
    post-assault sex focusing on, 2–3
    sex ed on, 54, 55, 132, 136, 139
    testing partners' respect for, 140–142
    withdrawing, 79, 137–140, 144, 183
containment, 31–32, 75
control, 118–120, 152, 162, 179, 180, 184, 198, 203
co-regulation, 60
C-PTSD. *See* complex post-traumatic stress disorder
CSA. *See* childhood sexual abuse
cuckolding, 197–199

Danielle (survivor), 124
dating, 4–5, 10, 31, 36, 43, 57, 65, 87, 95–96, 106, 127, 140, 164, 173, 201, 205. *See also* relationships with partners
deep pelvic breathing, 66
demisexuality, 53
Department of Veterans Affairs, 217
depression, 3, 200–204
desire for sex, 52–53, 125, 141, 191–192, 195–196
dirty talk, 164–165
disclosure of trauma history, 5, 6, 87–112, 131, 169, 201, 214
    aftercare on topic of, 210–211
    consent and, 137–138, 145
    in difficult and vulnerable conversations, 102–107
    for healthy, safe, pleasurable sex, 90–92
    involving abusive relationships, 19–20
    negative responses to, 88–90, 96–97, 107–111
    for normalization, 88
    as process, 99–100, 102–103, 112
    as root of fantasy, 85–86
    situations not requiring, 105–107, 111
    and STI status, 194
    to strangers vs. partners/friends, 92–102
    surface or summary, 99–100, 102
    survivor's control over, 108–110

timing of, 91–92, 97–98, 104, 111
and triggers, 148, 165
dissociation, 3, 8, 48, 56, 83, 84, 99–100, 149,
152–154, 161, 163, 165, 166, 178, 181,
193
domestic violence. *See* abusive relationships
dominance (dominant role), 46–47, 77, 104,
167, 170–171, 198
Down With Love (TV series), 139

Elsa (survivor), 76
embodied consent, 131–132, 137, 141–143,
165, 166, 210
embodied sex, 79, 160
embodied symptoms of trauma, 194–195
EMDR (eye movement desensitization and
reprocessing therapy), 74, 155
empathy, 15, 88, 92, 106, 132, 203, 212
erotica, 82
experimentation, 156–161
exposure therapy, 36
eye movement desensitization and
reprocessing therapy (EMDR), 74, 155

fantasies, 77–86
based on written vs. visual media, 81–83
disclosing traumatic root of, 85–86
flashbacks and nightmares vs., 78–79
for healing, 80–82
as others' triggers, 77–79, 83–84
post-trauma shifts in, 80
pressure to act out partner's, 197–198
in relationships with partners, 83–85
scripts and protocols for, 156–157
fear response, 10–11, 30, 153, 167, 214
fertility issues, 190–191, 195
fetish, 150–152, 165–169. *See also specific types*
Fifty Shades of Grey series, 168
fight or flight response, 3, 18, 185
first dates, 95–96, 106
first post-assault relationships, 99–101, 108–
109, 118–119, 126–128, 197–199
first post-assault sexual experience, 2–4,
113–129
beginner's mindset in, 124
healing in rebounds, 121–123
impact of trauma on, 113–115, 125
mind–body connection in, 128–129
pleasure in, 180–181

for survivors in relationships, 123–128
timing of, 128–129
triggers in, 152–155
and views of virginity, 115–117
vulnerability and shame in, 117–121
first relationships, abusive, 25–26
first sexual experience, assault as, 117
flashbacks, 8, 37, 78, 83, 85, 100, 149
fraternities, 44
freeze or appease response, 3, 18–19, 48, 125, 156
friends
disclosing trauma history to, 97, 98, 100,
102, 112
former partners as, 199, 213–216
sex with, 4, 106–107, 124, 213–214
support from, 19–21, 59, 67–69, 76, 202,
210–211
future-oriented healing, 28, 41

gaslighting, 14, 41, 60, 111, 162, 214
gay survivors. *See* LGBTQ+ survivors
gender identity stereotypes, 44–45
gender norms, 167–168
ghosting, 60, 199
Gomez, Gabby (survivor), 27, 74, 112, 152,
154–157, 165
"good girl" role, 47
grooming, 73
grounding, 169–170
group sex, 150

healing, 5, 59–76
aftercare for, 213–216
consent and, 142
disclosure and, 88–89, 98–99, 103
fantasies for, 80–82
feeling "healed," 203
in first post-assault sexual experience, 181
in friendships, 67–69
in health-care settings, 71–73
identity-related issues with, 61–62
and influences on behavior, 47
in isolation, 69–71
language for, 60–61
masturbation and, 178–179
open communication in, 75–76
in post-assault sexual experiences, 125
as priority, 35
in rebound relationships, 120–123

healing (*cont.*)
    in relationships with partners, 62–66
    safety for, 13, 27–30
    setbacks and, 189–190
    sexual education for, 39–41, 45–46
    social support for, 210
    in therapy, 66–67, 73–75
    triggers and, 148, 153–154
health-care settings, 42, 71–73, 117, 175–178,
    194–195, 200–201
Herman, Judith, 73–74
Hinge, 120
hookups, 30, 50, 76, 84–85, 95–96, 98, 105,
    114–115, 120, 125–126, 131–132,
    134, 136–138, 143, 148, 180–181, 183,
    202–205. *See also* casual sex
hunting play, 170–171
hyperarousal, 14, 83, 149
hypercompartmentalization, 69
hypersexuality, 200

identity issues, 49–54
infidelity, 17–19, 191–192, 206
intergenerational silence, 6
intimate partner violence. *See* abusive
    relationships
intuitive eating, 49, 66
isolation, 3, 45–46, 69–71, 174, 176, 183, 200,
    204, 210
IUD insertion, 177

Jennifer (survivor), 13, 27, 111–112

kink, 47, 57, 81, 124, 136–137, 150–152,
    159–160, 162, 165–170, 209. *See also*
    specific types
Kinsey Institute, 218
kissing, 118, 148, 193

laughter, as love language, 182
Laura (survivor), 52–53, 66, 141–142, 195–196
Lee, Leanna (survivor), 30–31, 35–36, 53, 56–
    57, 62–63, 68–69, 81–83, 99–102, 124,
    144, 151, 184–185, 192–193, 210–212
lesbian survivors. *See* LGBTQ+ survivors
Lexi M. (survivor), 11–12, 31–32, 36–37, 48–
    49, 51, 53–54, 60, 66–67, 78–79, 98–99,
    103–106, 134–136, 139, 156, 164–165,
    169–171, 189–190, 196–200

LGBTQ+ survivors
    bisexuality, 54, 69, 71
    consent for, 134–135
    cultural misunderstandings about, 149
    disclosure and coming out for, 5, 96–98
    identity exploration for, 4–5, 33–35, 49–50,
        62
    identity shifts and questioning for, 51–54,
        212
    play parties as safe spaces for, 136
    sexual education deficit for, 40
Libby (survivor), 25–27
libido. *See* desire for sex
long-distance relationships, 209
Lorde, Audre, 160
love bombing, 60

mania, 200–201
manipulation, 108, 111, 126, 132, 195–196
marginalized groups, 73–74, 162. *See also*
    LGBTQ+ survivors; people of color
Marin, Vanessa, 162
marriage, 31, 52–53, 81, 90–91, 99–101, 111,
    125, 135, 141–142, 144, 153–154, 182,
    184–185, 191–192, 195–197, 206, 215
masculinity, 44–47, 96–97
masking, 105
Mason (survivor), 15, 45–46, 69–71, 84–86,
    96–98, 106, 164, 166–167, 181–182,
    203–204, 211, 215
massage, 66, 169, 195–196
masturbation, 2, 78, 116, 163, 178–180, 185
Matthew (survivor), 49–50, 54, 75, 80, 106,
    112, 134–135, 142, 149, 164, 183
media representations, 42–46, 57–58, 82–83,
    94–95, 197
medical professionals, 42, 71–72, 117, 175–
    178, 194–195, 200–201
meningitis, 194
mental illness, 51, 193, 200–201. *See also*
    specific types
#MeToo movement, 1, 6, 95, 133, 205
Mia (survivor), 22–24, 50, 52, 55–56, 61–62,
    102–103, 141, 181, 200, 212
microaggressions, 14, 205
mind–body connection, 128–129
mindfulness, 70, 85, 161
mixed episodes, bipolar, 200–201
mixed signals, 144

monogamy, 43, 81
Murray, Lyndsey (survivor), 50–51, 60–61, 64, 66, 90–92, 110–111, 126–128, 135, 148, 180, 185, 206

National Domestic Violence Hotline, 21, 217
National Sexual Violence Resources Center, 217
needs, 144–145, 173–174, 216
nightmares, 78–79, 136, 214
non-concordance, 175
nonmonogamy, 104, 150, 170, 197–199
nonsexual situations
    abusive, 12–13, 75
    aftercare in, 213–216
    pleasure from, 170–171
    triggers in, 163–164
    turn-ons in, 170–171
normalization of experience, 7–8, 27, 57–58, 71, 88, 95, 148, 212
"no," saying, 24–25, 51, 76, 104, 125, 133–135, 138, 139, 152, 193, 205
numbing creams, 178

Ocean, Frank, 71
October 7th massacre, 11
OMGYES, 218
1in6 (organization), 218
one-night stands, 79, 81, 114, 138, 159, 201. See also casual sex
online communities and forums, 20, 168–169, 176
open relationships, 53–54, 191–192
oral sex, 34, 84–85, 114, 148, 176–177, 182, 185, 193, 204
orgasm, 81, 180, 182–186

pain, 7, 8, 44–45, 72, 116, 131–132, 150–151, 173–178, 185, 194–195
panic attacks, 3, 4, 8, 37, 81, 83, 100, 108, 124, 128, 148, 150, 151, 154–155
partner(s). See also relationships with partners
    compassionate, 3, 4, 154
    conflict with, as trigger, 163
    consent from, 142–146
    control over, 51
    criteria for choosing, 67–68, 91–92, 101, 110, 187–189, 206–207
    disclosing trauma history to, 88–104, 107–111, 153

disclosing triggers to, 148–150
finding the "right," 153–154
friendships with former, 199, 213–216
giving pleasure to, 47, 181–182, 211
"ideal," 49, 80
performance for benefit of, 195–196
physically intimidating, 13–15
in rebound relationships, 121–122
respecting boundaries of, 144–145, 211
"safe," 10, 28–31, 53, 90–91
scripts/protocols for, 156
with sexual trauma histories, 52, 97
supportive, 28–29, 59–60, 64, 65, 157–158
teaching, to respond, 92
testing potential, 140–142
trustworthy, 165
trying to understand, 176–177
view of boundaries, 135–136
women's responsibility for, 116–117
party culture, 159
pathologization, 42, 145
pause, taking a, 79, 128, 131, 135, 137–138, 140, 143, 144, 152, 155, 157, 169
penetrative sex, 114–115, 117, 175–177
people of color, 14, 22–23, 50, 61–62
people pleasing, 105, 198–199
"perfect" victim, 18, 108
physical attraction, 5, 33, 40, 49, 53–54, 85–86, 120–123, 125–126, 150, 161–162, 200
physical health issues, 18–19, 51, 194–195, 200–201
physical safety, 12, 27, 214
Planned Parenthood, 39, 133, 217, 218
play parties, 136–137, 145–146
pleasure, 2–3, 90–92, 155–158, 169–170. See also turn-ons
    in broader definition of sex, 166–167
    centering, 176–178, 182–184
    in consensual encounters that resemble assault, 147, 149–150
    in hookups, 180–181
    masturbation for, 178–180
    and #MeToo movement, 6
    orgasm as goal of sex vs., 182–186
    with pain, 150–151. See also kink
    partners', 47, 181–182, 211
    in play dealing with triggers, 170–171
    positive consent for, 133–134
    regaining trust to experience, 181

polyamorous community, 170

pornography, 38, 54–55, 80, 82, 83

post-assault sexual experiences. *See also
        specific types*

on anniversary of assault, 164

diversity of, 6–7

effect of negative, 203–208

healthy, safe, pleasurable, 90–92, 155–158,
        169–170

multifaceted influences on, 45–48

normalizing, 7–8

"powering through," 152–153, 181

pressure to return to sex, 66

as project management, 77

shifts in fantasies, 80

trial-and-error approach to, 2–3

post-traumatic growth, 5–6

post-traumatic stress disorder (PTSD), 1, 3, 35,
        36, 56, 57, 62–63, 75, 83, 92, 124, 125,
        136, 147, 148, 164, 187, 193

power play, 105, 134

pregnancy, 13, 56, 62–63, 182, 190–193

present, being, 84–85, 143, 152, 184. *See also*
        mindfulness

primal dom, 170–171

promiscuous/prudish false binary, 42–43, 134,
        195

psychological control play, 156–157

psychological distress, 13, 202

Psychology Today, 218

PTSD. *See* post-traumatic stress disorder

purity culture, 55–56, 114–115

queer survivors. *See* LGBTQ+ survivors

quid pro quo, in dating, 140

radical acceptance, 85

Raimundo, Alicia (survivor), 48, 161–163,
        166, 168

Ramona (survivor), 13–15, 30, 53, 57–58, 64–
        66, 72–73, 95–96, 115–117, 142–144,
        167–168, 175–177, 183–185, 205

rape culture, 2, 6, 8, 13, 15–16, 22, 27, 30, 93

rape fantasies, 78, 79

rebound relationships, 120–123

recovery, 2, 5, 27–30, 117, 202

relationships with partners, 2–4. *See also*
        breakups; partners

abusive. *See* abusive relationships

aftercare for, 209–211

boundaries in, 50–53

consent in long-term, 139, 141–143

disclosure in, 87–88

fantasies in, 83–85

first post-assault sex in, 123–128

healing in, 59–60, 62–66, 70–71

internal struggles in, 101

masturbation and, 178–180

one-sided sex in, 158–159

orgasm as goal in, 182–186

pain during sex in, 173–178, 185–186

PTSD symptoms in, 56–57

rebound, 120–123

setbacks in, 192–193, 195, 206

sexual personas in, 46–48

socialized beliefs about, 197–199

triggers in, 153–156

turn-ons in, 151, 156–158, 165–166

resiliency, building up, 189

restraints, 81, 124, 151

revictimization, 201–208

"risky" sex, 42, 159, 200

Rivera, Ignacio G. (survivor), 27, 40–41, 84,
        88, 136–137, 144–146, 165, 202–203,
        209–210

role models, 61–62

role-playing, 80, 150. *See also* play parties

romance writing, 81–82, 102, 140

Rose, Stacey (survivor), 16–19, 21, 29, 38–39,
        44, 55, 68, 71, 74–75, 88–90, 92–95,
        121–123, 132–133, 180–182, 205

rough sex, 156–157, 204

safer sex, 57–58, 127–128, 146, 165

safe spaces, 13, 32, 91, 145–146

safety, 9–32, 79, 81

during breakups, 199

circumstantial threats to, 11–15

consent and, 136, 138, 145–146

and containment, 31–32

disclosure without, 90–91, 111

in first post-assault experiences, 122

for healing and recovery, 27–30

healthy, safe, pleasurable sexual experi-
        ences, 90–92, 155–158, 169–170

and impact of staying with abusers, 21–27

orgasm and, 184–185
physical, 12, 27, 214
"safe" partners, 10, 28–31, 53, 90–91
social support and, 19–21
for survivors in abusive relationships, 15–27
for triggered partner, 156
validation of boundaries for, 170
safewords, 140, 162, 165, 171
SAR (Sexual Attitudes Reassessment), 39
scripts, 156–157
second responders, 88–89
self-compassion, 44, 203
self-conception, 27, 41
self-worth, 50, 84, 135, 158, 200
setbacks for survivors, 187–208
breakups, 187–189, 196–200
fertility issues, 190–191
and healing, 189–190
infidelity, 191–192
in marriage, 195–196
medical, 194–195, 200–201
pregnancy, 192–193
revictimization, 201–208
sex, defining, 114, 115
sex education, 33, 37–42, 45–46, 50, 54–58, 132, 136, 139, 218
sex positivity, 55, 74, 155, 168
sexual agency, 25, 38, 41–42, 46, 61, 62, 158–160, 171, 186, 203, 205
sexual assault
anniversary of, 164
defining consent in reaction to, 138–140
experiencing more than one, 201–208
identity as someone who is experiencing, 64–66
minimizing experience of, 11–12, 24, 68–69, 73
negative consensual sex vs., 205
turn-ons in encounters that resemble, 147, 149–150
sexual assault survivors. See also specific topics
aftercare outside of sex for, 213–216
centering experience of, 212
issues specific to male, 44–45
judgment of, 17–19
with marginalized identities, 73–74, 162
resources for, 217–219
stereotypes about, 42–45, 61, 134

Sexual Attitudes Reassessment (SAR), 39, 55
sexual content, in entertainment, 46, 57. See also pornography
sexual exploration, 49–50, 53, 80, 113–114, 138, 150–151, 156–161, 184–185, 206–208, 210
sexual healing. See healing
sexual health information, 218
sexually transmitted infections (STIs), 194
Sexual preferences. See turn-ons
sexual prenup, 141
sexual self, 60–61
"sex vacations," 25, 152
shame, 43–44, 80, 109, 117–121, 148–150, 153, 159, 161–165, 177, 180, 183–184, 194, 196, 202, 204
"shoulds," 48, 85, 173, 177–178, 201
Simon, Katie (survivor), 1–8, 10–11, 33–36, 42–43, 47–48, 51, 59, 67, 75–78, 82, 83, 85–87, 90, 92, 100–102, 106–108, 110, 111, 113–115, 118–121, 125–126, 128–129, 131–132, 134, 148, 150, 163, 164, 173–174, 177–180, 187–189, 200–202, 206–208, 210–215
slapping, 170
sleeping around. See casual sex
slutty phases. See casual sex
social support, 19–21, 59–60, 66–67, 210–216. See also healing; partners, supportive; support groups
somatics, 31–32, 36–37, 169, 189
statutory rape, 25–27
stigma, 13, 43, 44, 98, 109, 194
stopping, 79, 137–140, 144, 183
strangers, disclosing history to, 92
submissive role, 47, 77, 167
substance use, 198
suicidality, 202–204
Suicide and Crisis Lifeline, 217
support groups, 59, 76
surprises, 81, 82, 168, 211
survival skills, 63
Surviving R. Kelly (TV series), 94
survivor narratives
author's, 1–6
diversity of, 5–8
need for, 8
switch, BDSM, 160

Talkspace, 218
talk therapy, 66, 102
tend and befriend response. *See* freeze or
    appease response
therapy, 2, 5, 28, 63, 66–67, 73–75, 103, 141,
    155, 158, 162, 192–193, 198–199, 206,
    218
threesomes, 104
throwaway sex, 119–120
Title IX programs, 16, 38
titration, somatic, 169
touch, as trigger, 118, 139, 142–143, 181
transgender survivors. *See* LGBTQ+ survivors
trauma, 2, 12, 27, 63, 70
    compounding, 62–63
    distancing self from, 193
    embodied symptoms of, 194–195
    impact of, on first post-assault sexual
        experience, 113–115, 125
    for male survivors, 44–45
    partners' ability to navigate, 187–189
    persistence of, 35–36, 153–154, 189
    sexual education and ability to navigate,
        54–58
trauma bonding, 90
trauma-sensitive dating, 3
traumatic stress, 3, 24, 29
Trevor Project, The, 218
triggers, 36–37, 57, 63, 75
    addressing, for safe and pleasurable sex,
        155–158, 169–170
    audio, 93, 163
    changes in, 149–151
    circumstantial, 163–164
    containment of, 31–32
    defined, 147
    disclosing/communicating about, 91,
        93–95, 100, 104, 107, 110, 148, 149,
        155, 169
    in first post-assault relationship, 117, 124
    helping survivors reengage after, 165
    in initial post-assault sex, 152–155
    nonsexual, 93–94, 100, 163–164
    others' fantasies as, 77–79, 83–84
    pain as, 175, 177

play related to dealing with, 170–171
    relationships between sex acts and,
        147–149
    somatic view of, 189
    turn-ons and, 147, 149, 157
    unwanted sex as, 195–196
trust, 104–106, 118, 144, 151, 161, 177, 181,
    206
turn-ons
    changes in, 150–151, 171
    communication about, 104, 128, 149–150,
        165–170
    consent and, 132, 134, 141
    discussing, with triggers and trauma
        history, 169
    experimenting with, 156–161
    exploration to discover, 150–151
    kink and fetish as, 150–152, 165–169
    masturbation, 180
    in nonsexual situations, 170–171
    preferred roles, 46–48
    in relationships with partners, 151, 156–
        158, 165–166
    triggers and, 147, 149, 157
    values and, 161–163

vaginismus, 72, 175
validation, 212
values, 161–163, 194, 198
vanilla sex, 77, 79, 81, 137, 166, 167, 195
vibrators, 179
victim blaming, 66
violation, threat of, 1–2
violent content, on television, 82–83
virginity, 115–117, 119
vulnerability, 91, 93, 96, 102–107, 117–121,
    138, 183

weapons, 79
WomensLaw, 217
written materials, 81–82, 102, 140

Xanax, 153

yoni massage, 66

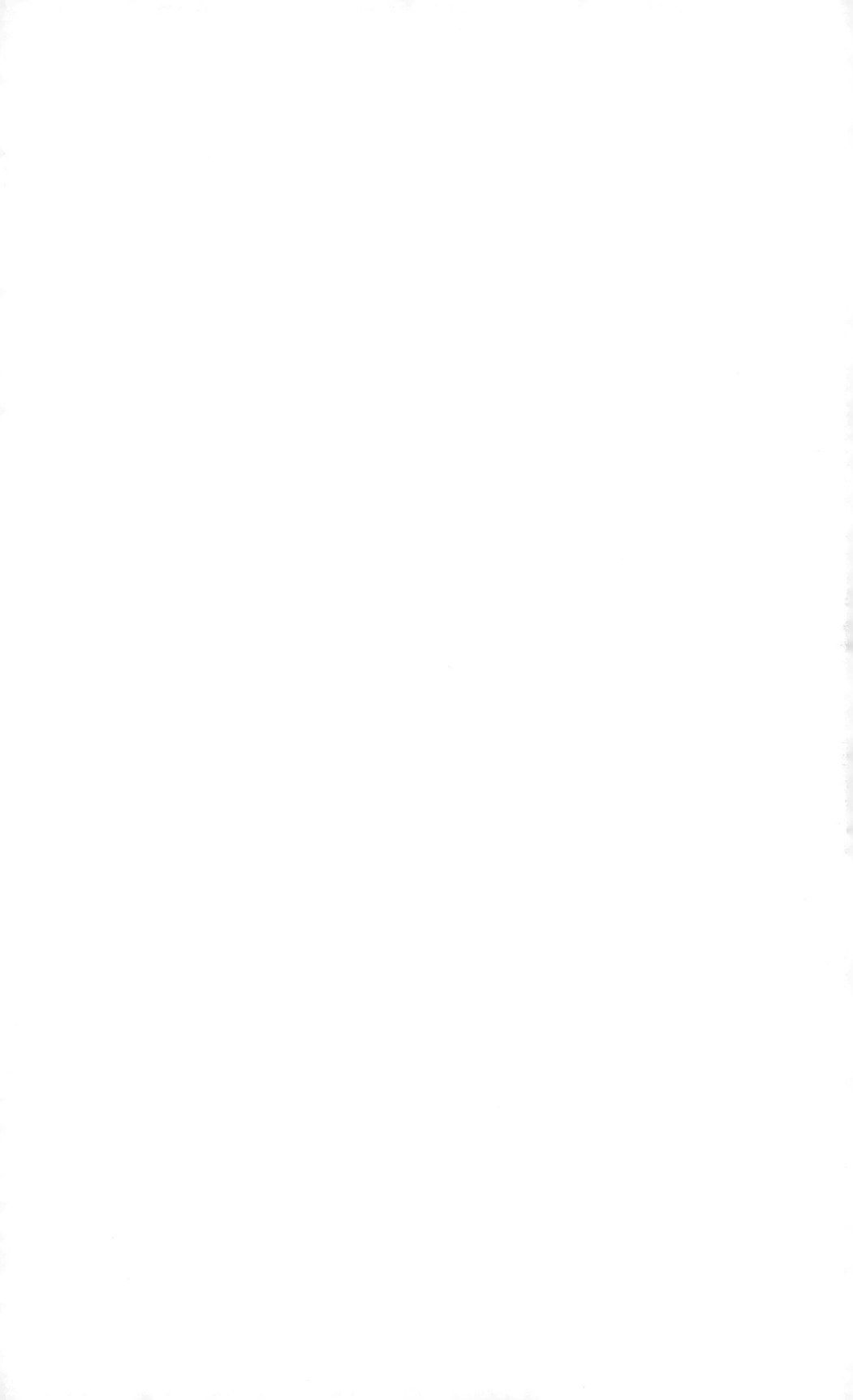

01 14